STOP

FEMALE GENITAL MUTILATION

WOMEN SPEAK

FACTS AND ACTIONS

FRAN P. HOSKEN

PUBLISHED BY: WOMEN'S INTERNATIONAL NETWORK NEWS.
187 GRANT STREET, LEXINGTON, MA 02173. USA

ISBN 0-942096-10-X

TABLE OF CONTENTS

PUBLISHED BY: WOMEN'S INTERNATIONAL NETWORK NEWS.
187 GRANT STREET, LEXINGTON, MA 02173. USA

PREFACE

This book is based on the fourth edition of **The HOSKEN REPORT: Genital and Sexual Mutilation of Females,** published in January 1994, in which the extensive research summarized here is documented and detailed. **The HOSKEN REPORT** is the most comprehensive research work on Female Genital Mutilation (FGM), providing case histories of 10 African countries (Sudan, Egypt, Kenya, Somalia, Ethiopia, Mali, Nigeria, Burkina Faso, Sierra Leone and Senegal) and a history of FGM. A global overview of FGM is given, including Asia and the Western world, as well as a 12-page bibliography.

In this book, the key chapter "Women Speak About Their Lives" relates the personal stories of women from all over Africa. Most of these accounts are told by the women themselves, describing their own experiences. The stories were gathered over many years from many different sources. These very personal histories, from different regions and very different African societies, shed some light on the social conditions and family life that so greatly influence and often determine girls' and women's lives and health over which they still have very little control - and that must change.

Though these personal stories are told by women living thousands of miles apart, **they are bound together by a common fate and by a shared experience imposed on them - the mutilation of their bodies and lives.** What was done to these women makes them victims of their patriarchal societies and environment, which up to now most women have been quite unable to change, though this is now beginning to be questioned.

To take control of our lives and to reach out beyond the narrow limits imposed on us in societies ruled by men, is a yearning that women share everywhere in the world. It is a goal we shall and must achieve for our children, and this is what this book is all about - **the need for change!** The demand for recognition of our human rights is growing louder everywhere. **This fundamental social revolution is bringing women together and gaining all over the world.**

As this book goes to press, on the eve of the **United Nations Fourth World Conference on Women in Beijing,** more and more women are beginning to take control of their own bodies and lives and, with it, their future. I hope that what is reported here will convince all who read it to join together in working for a new, free, open, and equal way of life.

Finally, I want to thank all the women whose stories are related here, the many others who have made this book possible, and especially those who have supported my work.

Fran P. Hosken
Lexington, Massachusetts, USA
August 1995

INTRODUCTION

It is 22 years since I first began to work against female genital mutilation (FGM), an African practice that was unknown at that time in most of the world. Some background facts need to be summarized, based on this experience, to provide some context and to relate to our own lives what is reported here. When I discovered the existence of FGM, after having traveled widely on all other continents, very few facts were recorded and the dimension of the problem was unknown. Rather, as I soon began to discover, information on FGM was deliberately concealed or misrepresented, especially by international organizations including United Nations agencies and church groups working in Africa.

I learned about FGM in 1973, on my first research trip to 15 countries and 25 cities in sub-Saharan Africa, while reporting on urbanization, housing and building - my professional fields - and researching women's development. At the beginning of the trip in Kenya I learned for the first time about FGM in a casual conversation with a young English woman working in Nairobi. I asked about her work, about her Kenyan contemporaries and friends, and she quite graphically and openly described what she had learned.

It was hard to believe that such practices exist today, so I began to ask more questions. Was this a local practice, was it done in other parts of Africa, why and by whom? Though I tried to get more information throughout this trip, where I met with many African women's organizations, it was impossible to get any reliable facts. There was a wall of silence and denial surrounding this issue. I did not realize until much later that the only place to get the facts was at maternity hospitals and by talking to the midwives. No published information on FGM was available in Africa at that time

"How did you discover FGM, and why did you get involved?" is the question I am most frequently asked every time I speak on the subject. Perhaps the best answer is another question: **how could I not get involved,** once I found out what it was all about? How can you walk past a mutilated dying child in the street and do nothing, or pretend you did not see? How can you work for women's rights - I first learned about FGM when International Women's Year was just beginning to be discussed all over the world - and ignore the deliberate violation of millions of girls and women? It seemed to me the height of hypocrisy to prepare for **the first-ever global conference on women in 1975 and a year of international activities by and for women around the world,** while ignoring what still was called then "female circumcision" - a verbal disguise to conceal the reality.

Or, as so many repeatedly told me, **"This is an African tradition and an African affair, therefore it can't be touched and is of no concern to the rest of the world."** But this most widely used excuse for failing to protect girls and women has always been unacceptable to me and, now also, to all concerned with women's and human rights.

It took me some time to realize and comprehend the terrible truth about what was really being done to the bodies of little girls. I simply could not believe it at first; how could anyone even think up such a dreadful way to torture a child? But then I learned about the permanent lifelong consequences of what these children were subjected to and how FGM distorts all the rest of their lives with repeated, debilitating suffering. **Why? Why would anyone do such a terrible thing and then make it into a regular practice to which all girl children were subjected?** What do people really gain from this? This question I am still unable to answer, especially since so many millions of children are involved.

I was so shaken by what I learned that I knew I had to find the truth. Initially I hoped that this was not really happening, or that such practices were isolated and disappearing, as so many tried to tell me when I began to investigate. **The first task, therefore, was to establish the facts on where FGM was practiced - why, by whom and how many people were affected - before it was possible to break the silence and bring the problem to the attention of the world in order to do something about it.**

When I returned from Africa I started a systematic investigation; I spent much time at medical libraries, wrote hundreds of letters and sent questionnaires on maternal health all over Africa. I wrote to health and social development ministries of all African governments as well as to hundreds of international nongovernmental organizations (NGOs) working in mother and child health and population in connection with the planned International Women's Year.

It was incredibly difficult to get any reliable information. Both the World Health Organization (WHO) and UNICEF refused to help, claiming they were protecting "African culture and tradition" (see chapter on "Politics"). For years I pieced together information from all different sources scattered all over the world. I collected all published medical articles and wrote to their authors for more information. It was not only difficult to find the truth, **but some traditional international organizations reacted with surprising hostility, attacking me for being an American feminist, which was used as a pejorative at the time by patriarchal international organizations.** I was not inexperienced - I had lived on two continents, had an excellent professional education, raised a family and had traveled extensively all over the world, reporting for several international papers besides teaching and publishing several books. My knowledge of several languages helped to bring the widely scattered published information together which had never been done before.

Finally, in response to my inquiries sent to African governments, **the minister of social affairs of Sudan, Dr. Fatma Mahmoud, a gynecologist by profession** and the only woman in the Government, sent me the most comprehensive clinical study of FGM ever made. **This research, published in Sudan by Dr. Abu el Futuh Shandall, is still the most comprehensive investigation on FGM: the facts documented and published there cannot be denied,** as so many I contacted tried to do. It was a critical breakthrough for my work.

From the start, when I first heard about FGM in Nairobi, I was determined to find the truth, which turned out to be not only elusive but scattered all over Africa. The fact that FGM is practiced in such a huge region was unknown. I had to gradually assemble and carefully check each piece of information to determine the dimensions of the problem, including how many girls and women are affected. **These essential facts were not only hidden in Africa by Africans directly involved (there were no African publications on FGM except the research in Khartoum),** but the European and North American organizations working in Africa, including missionaries, health care and development professionals, seemed to deliberately ignore the systematic mutilation of millions of little girls.

Why would the professional staff of United Nations agencies, especially UNICEF and WHO which are concerned with children and health, continue to conceal FGM for so many years? This conspiracy of silence had the support of most international NGOs and church groups of every denomination. All this is further discussed in the chapter on "Politics." Most of these organizations are headed, organized and run by men, and all decisions regarding international matters are made by men to this day.

Most of the highly financed development and population programs that today work in Africa and the Middle East, where the vast majority of girl children continue to be mutilated, **do nothing effective even now to prevent such child assault. Yet FGM goes on in their very program areas with the knowledge of those who run projects** concerned with family planning and reproductive health. For instance, a family health program advisor working for the Canadian Government told me she was honored to be invited to an excision ceremony. **Did she try to provide the families involved with health information on the health damage done by FGM?** I asked. "But we cannot interfere," she replied.

The same code - an international conspiracy of silence - prevailed all over the world on WIFE ABUSE AND FAMILY VIOLENCE BY MEN AGAINST FEMALE FAMILY MEMBERS. AND THAT IS THE FIRST CRITICAL ISSUE TO EXAMINE HERE.

WIN NEWS which I started in 1975 has reported regularly on violence by men against women from a global perspective since 1977, when wife abuse first began to surface after centuries of silence. I have recorded how, from its slow start, the discussion of male violence against women and children began to be taken up by women worldwide. **Women now are speaking up and protesting the destructive attacks by men against women of their own families which goes on** everywhere in the world. Hidden by silence it was protected by the patriarchal family structure that oppresses women everywhere.

By now, wife abuse and violence by men against female family members and FGM are regularly reported as human rights violations in the annually published **Country Reports on Human Rights Practices** by the Department of State. In 1994, the reports covered 193 countries. (See every spring issue of **WIN NEWS**.) I started lobbying Congress and the State Department to include FGM and wife abuse in these annual reports during the Carter Administration in the 1970's. For years I have been providing the State Department country team leaders who prepare these reports with information on women and FGM, **which is now reported in every African country where practiced and locally documented. But in every country world-wide, without exception, abuse and killing of female family members by family men is reported; it is a universal feature of the patriarchal system.**

As with FGM, the denial of the existence of male abuse of female family members was and is persistent. **Much like FGM, wife abuse is also regarded as a "hallowed tradition" and "cultural right" by many men all over the world.** Both wife abuse and FGM are conclusively documented and can no longer be denied: everywhere these violent practices are **taught from father to son in the patriarchal family, where "might is right."**

Extensive media and public campaigns to stop male violence against women have been and continue to be organized by women all over the world. Slowly and reluctantly they are being joined by health departments in some countries, because of the hospitalization costs incurred by so many injured women. Even WHO, the most conservative male-dominated global health system, had to recently admit that **the largest source of injuries to women globally is violence by men!** Judicial systems are becoming reluctantly involved as there are more women judges now as well as police - though it is widely documented that policemen beat their own wives much like all other men. All this, and more, is reported regularly in **the section on violence in WIN NEWS.**

Recently the cover-up of wife abuse was again being promoted by US politicians who deplore that so many women are single heads of families. **Yet FBI statistics show that more women are injured and killed by their husband or "lovers" than in car accidents.** Instead of protecting women, the US legislators propose to cancel financial help for children of single mothers to force women back into patriarchal families headed by abusive men. A researcher recently stated on television that **during a recent eight-year period as many women were killed by their men as US soldiers died in Vietnam.** Around the world one-third of families are headed by women - **and one reason is male violence.**

While actions against wife abuse in many parts of the world are slowly being initiated due to relentless work by women demanding protection and change, actions against FGM are greatly hampered not only by misogynist attitudes but by pervasive racial prejudice on both sides. **FGM is an indigenous African ethnic practice that originated in Africa and is widespread today among sub-Saharan and Middle Eastern population groups.** It is essential that the eradication of FGM is never confused with discrimination. **How can we tolerate the mutilation of a female child just because she is brown or black? This is racism at its worst - and a violation of human rights.**

THE NEXT CRITICAL ISSUE THAT NEEDS TO BE EXAMINED IS THE RESPONSIBILITY FOR FGM BY MEN. This is not reverse discrimination but it is a fact that cannot be denied after many years of investigation, and it finally must be faced or nothing will really change. First of all, **men are in control of everything in Africa, especially of women and children who are wholly owned property of men.** Women have no legal power and few legal rights which they cannot enforce. They are excluded from all political power on the national and community level as well as from decision making in their patriarchal families.

Women are excluded from owning land, the chief resource in all the predominantly agricultural African societies. By tradition they are denied all property rights. They are sold into marriage by their fathers for a brideprice in cash or kind; there is no alternative but marriage for every woman in Africa, though she has no say in the deal. **FGM is a marriage requirement demanded by men,** therefore the practice continues. **It is as simple as that. If tomorrow African men were to publicly declare they will not marry mutilated brides, FGM would stop.** As long as men do not, FGM will continue on a continent where marriage for a woman is essential since by tradition she has no rights of her own. A woman is part of a patriarchal polygamous family ruled by men.

To be sure, the facts stated here apply to the vast majority of the mostly rural African women and not the tiny minority who come to international gatherings or the few that study at Western universities. These privileged women are highly educated and lead sophisticated, internationally influenced lives. If their husbands and **the men of their families who are the leaders of Africa - political, military, religious and business - would publicly declare that their sons will not take brides who are excised or infibulated the practice would stop.** But to set such an example with their own families takes real leadership, which so far African men have quite failed to demonstrate.

In this summary of the extensive research published in **The HOSKEN REPORT** and especially in the new chapter on **Women Speak About Their Lives,** it becomes clear why these mutilations continue to be performed: because they are demanded by the vast majority of African men. **But what is critical is that men from all other countries who work in Africa, in solidarity with African men, never speak about FGM: their silence supports FGM.** Yes, the operators who actually do the mutilations are mostly women simply because women have no choice. Women have been subservient to men for generations. Most women in Africa have no life of their own outside their families. Rather, women are dependent members of families that are headed by men who make all the rules.

The vast majority of women in Africa and the Middle East cannot read or write, they live in polygamous households and are engaged all their lives in childbearing, childrearing and growing food on their husbands' land to feed their families. Their daily household tasks require the hardest manual labor. Their education is from their mothers and grandmothers. They are socialized in their polygamous traditional families and raised with customs from the past. It was always that way. The mutilation of all female children is "natural"; it is decreed by the ancestors. A terrible fate is in store for those who do not follow tradition. **No man will marry a girl who is intact, and that is critical: there is no choice, all daughters are "done."** To make it acceptable and hide the horrible reality the mutilations in many places are disguised by celebrations and loud noise to cover up the shrieks of the little victims. In some areas not even that kind of disguise is used, or else the victims are taken outside the village to suffer in isolation removed from all support.

The stark reality shown here in the collected stories of women from all over Africa, is that the victims involved simply have no alternative; they are children and never asked. Their mothers do not know that any other way of life is possible or that women in most of the world are not mutilated in this terrible way. As the stories of the women show, **FGM is always presented as an essential part of each woman's life.** For a person who has no contact beyond her village and community, who cannot read or knows no language but her local dialect, who has no human connection with the strange world outside, the very idea of change is unknown, or worse, anything new is threatening.

Urbanization - the move into towns, which implies a radical change in lifestyle - is creating enormous new problems on a continent that lacks most infrastructure and basic services such as water supply, sewers, electricity and roads. Originally I went to Africa to study and report on urbanization, housing and building, my professional field. Africa is now urbanizing faster than any other continent. That means rural people are moving into towns unable to deal with the newcomers, who squat on every available piece of land without water supply or any way to support themselves.

But women are the last ones to leave the rural areas in Africa to go to live in towns or move to an urban environment. Mostly men go alone, leaving their families, wives and children behind to fend for themselves. Men learn something new in town. **Women stay physically and mentally behind, cut off from all innovation and change.** Men come home to father more children and make the decisions about their land, which is farmed by their women to grow the food for their many children in traditional laborious ways.

According to tradition, women in most of Africa have no rights to the land and no rights to the houses where they live, no rights to the crops they grow and no rights to their own children. It is the father who decides to whom his daughters are given in marriage in return for the brideprice paid to him: all decisions are made among men. As long as men refuse to marry women who are not mutilated according to local custom, the mutilations will continue. **FGM will go on until women have established, assured and confirmed rights to own property and, with this, their own bodies and lives - independent of men.**

The real dilemma that women confront was brought home at a meeting on FGM at the medical school in Mogadishu the first time I visited Somalia, in 1979, upon invitation of the Somali delegation to the Khartoum seminar on "Traditional Practices Affecting the Health of Women and Children," organized by WHO. This meeting, organized by Somali leaders committed to change, was held to publicize the international recommendations to eradicate FGM formulated in Khartoum. I was invited to present the global review of FGM as I had done at the seminar.

A large group of midwives - dressed in white, as is traditional - attended the meeting as they handle all births in that country. **During the question period a midwife stood up and asked the physicians and officials: "Tell me what am I to do.** I have several daughters, one is reaching the age where the operations are usually done. As a midwife I know from my own experience the terrible problems that result in childbirth due to infibulation - and every woman I deliver has had this operation. I know the terrible pain, the bleeding, the injuries that often result. I can't have this done to my own child. But if I don't she will never find a husband; **no man will want to marry her and her life will be ruined. She will blame me. Why didn't I have her operated? She will hate me because she will become an outcast, unmarried, without children and rejected by all. Tell me, doctors, what am I to do?"**

As long as African men demand the mutilations as price for marriage and **these patriarchal traditions are supported by men around the world, this will continue. Why do men in the rest of the world fail to speak up? Why are physicians especially silent?** Why do the international programs in health and population continue to ignore the ongoing mutilations of millions of helpless girl children, now that all the facts are known? If they would all act together they soon could convince men in Africa that it is in their own interest to stop demanding FGM; no man is beyond learning the truth that **the prestige and status of men does not depend on mutilating women to assert their manhood, which is what their failure to stop FGM really means.**

Peer groups such as the many international professional groups of physicians and of both men and women working in different branches public health, as well as other international professional organizations, for instance, in education, have always worked together internationally in mutual support. Years ago I developed a program suggesting that such organizations **set up programs to work together to stop damaging practices and to improve health, including the local male leadership. Professional support groups have been successfully formed on many issues. Such peer groups of professionals for the abolishment of FGM could set an example** to the male leadership and provide support to isolated local groups by forming networks to encourage men to come forward. At the time I contacted professional groups there was no response: now that **the Inter-African Committee (IAC) on Traditional Practices has shown the way** it should be tried again.

THE THIRD INTERNATIONAL CONCERN THAT HAS BECOME A GROWING AND INCREASINGLY THREATENING ISSUE IS THE MEDICALIZATION OF FGM: the introduction of the mutilations into modern medical practice under the mistaken label to make FGM safer for women. How can a deliberate excision or mutilation of a functional healthy organ be safe? Yet this is the rhetoric that accompanies such posturing.

At the United Nations population conference in Cairo in September 1994, the issue of **FGM was repeatedly discussed at the Forum** - the NGO parallel meeting to the government conference. **An actual operation done in the home of a family in Cairo was videotaped and shown on cable television news worldwide during the conference.** The reaction to this damaging publicity, given the global audience at the conference, was a statement by the Egyptian president that legislation will be formulated, after he had previously claimed in an interview that FGM was not practiced in Egypt.

As soon as the conference participants left the real reaction set in, not only among the Islamic scholars, some of whom claimed that the Koran supports FGM while before they said the opposite, **but predictably physicians also spoke up, as a large source of income is involved.** In Egypt, midwives or dayas (traditional birth attendants) are prohibited from doing the operations, which leaves this lucrative field open for physicians who mostly operate on the daughters of the well-to-do among the urban population.

In an article published in the British Medical Journal of Jan. 7, 1995, a gynecologist at Cairo University, Dr. Munir Fawzi, in reaction to the discussion of legislation against FGM, is quoted in favor of the procedure; he **called on the Egyptian Government to support training programs for physicians to do the mutilations the medical way, under anesthesia. He offered to organize such training at his university.** He was joined by another prominent **Egyptian doctor who declared that no man would marry his daughters unless they were operated.** (See spring and summer issues of **WIN NEWS** 1995.)

That unfortunately confirms again that not only in sub-Saharan Africa but also in Egypt and the Middle East **the decisions about FGM are made exclusively by men or under the direction of men. Women are neither consulted nor asked, and most of the time** - as their own stories in the chapter on "Women Speak" show - the idea that women could resist, or have other ways to deal with their bodies, does not even occur to the men who discuss the medicalization of FGM under the oppressive climate of the patriarchal culture.

The medicalization of FGM, besides in Egypt, now goes on mainly in the capitals of most sub-Saharan African countries where FGM is traditionally practiced. This could not happen without the collusion of international medicine. The failure of WHO to promote the implementation of the 1979 WHO seminar recommendations has allowed medicalization of FGM to become a lucrative field literally everywhere in Africa. **Though WHO has representatives in every member country including all of Africa and the Middle East, these physicians, many of whom I visited, do not seem to be concerned about FGM or women's health.** Supported by the silence of all internationally funded health and especially the multimillion-dollar population programs that are currently going on all over Africa, medicalization is taking hold.

Most large population programs in Africa are funded by the US Agency for International Development (USAID) and by the World Bank: their contractors working in Africa refuse to even acknowledge the existence of FGM, which goes on under the noses of their highly paid international experts without any objection by anyone. FGM continues to be practiced even in the program areas of organizations that claim to teach women about reproductive health and family planning. The operations are being modernized and medicalized by the trained African program personnel as an income-generating sideline, using imported tools, imported antibiotics and the training in health provided at the program's expense.

Claiming deference to African culture and tradition, promoted by African men, thousands of little African girls are mutilated every year the "medical way" with US-supplied antibiotics, training and tools, with the collusion of US program directors and health experts and paid for by taxpayers' money. Most of the USAID health and population experts have never acknowledged that FGM exists. The WHO recommendations, which provide guidelines for action, have not been officially recognized, and the ongoing medicalization in AID-funded program areas has been ignored.

As recently documented in Kenya by the new program of the Maendeleo Ya Wanawake Organization (Women's Progress) to stop FGM, their investigations show that **in all four areas in Kenya where research was done the local hospitals do FGM for a fee** - which is higher than what local women excisors charge. **In Kenya, the ongoing mutilations of the genitalia of female children in hospitals including missionary hospitals was officially prohibited by President arap Moi in 1982.** This prohibition of FGM in Kenya was repeated several times since then. But the practice and its medicalization are condoned in all international population and health program areas.

When I visited the Abidjan office of a large population and health program run by Columbia University, one of the physicians working for the program whom I asked about FGM, which is practiced in the entire area, told me, **"This is a sacred practice and we certainly will not touch it."** When I informed the director of the program in New York and challenged him as a gynecologist to deal with the issue, as the health of millions of women was at risk, he told me he was not going to interfere. His reaction was quite typical of US physicians working in Africa and/or organizing African programs in population and health. **One can but wonder about the medical oath these men claim to take "to do no harm."** (See chapter on "Politics.")

The greatest danger at present is that FGM will be made into a medical procedure in urban areas where health services are available for those who can afford to pay for it. This will persuade politicians and decision makers that their daughters and families are taken care of: they need no longer fear losing the brideprice and the important political alliances that are fashioned by marriage due to the death of their girls as result of excision. Therefore any campaigns to stop these practices, which would upset their male political followers, are unnecessary and male domination remains secure and assured.

Outside interference never was a real threat as long as African men kept control over their families and polygamous households, and **they could count on the global patriarchal establishment as well as the support by patriarchal religion - especially the growing Moslem fundamentalists and the Catholic Church. Medicalization also eliminates interference by the international medical establishment** as it keeps local physicians and the health sector busy, well paid for their services and therefore free of protest.

For instance, in Mogadishu, before the program to develop a strategy to stop FGM was started by the SWDO (Somali Women's Democratic Organization), **the main hospital in Mogadishu had developed a program to infibulate little girls in the main operating rooms** once a week on a veritable production line. The parents who brought the girls paid at the door. Specially trained male nurses in gowns and masks did the operations and gave out antibiotics to be taken home to prevent infection. This was documented in detail in a medical article translated and published in **The HOSKEN REPORT.**

A British physician wrote to WIN NEWS a few years ago, asking me to publish about his great contribution of doing excisions safely the medical way, and he sent a detailed description. He had practiced this method in Sierra Leone, in the hospital in Freetown, as he became aware of the large number of severely injured girls brought in after being mutilated by the traditional matrons in the secret ceremonies in the Bundu Bush. As a global women's network **he expected WIN NEWS to praise him and publish his important contribution protecting the health of African girls and women!** (See chapter on "Politics.")

There are many more such stories: **but how can the consciousness of the patriarchal medical establishment be raised - especially those from the old school** now working internationally in decision-making positions. International medicine is mainly concerned with curative care addressing illness rather than keeping people healthy through preventive care. Childbirth is not an illness, and therefore has been ignored until quite lately by international medicine including WHO, despite 500,000 annual deaths by childbearing women - most of them preventable with simple precautions. Recent initiatives to reduce the scandalously high death rates due to pregnancy are mainly on paper, ignoring the most necessary actions in the field - especially in rural areas in Africa. **Maternal deaths due to pregnancy-related causes predictably are the highest in the world in Africa where FGM is practiced. Yet the fact that FGM is the cause is still deliberately ignored by the very physicians who claim to make childbirth safe.**

The failure of WHO to speak out against the medicalization of FGM since the 1979 seminar in Khartoum is in part responsible for its spread. WHO even omitted any mention of medicalization from the formal briefing on FGM held at the World Health Assembly in the spring of 1994. Each spring representatives of health ministries from all over the world come together in Geneva to discuss global health policies. The briefing on FGM included a presentation by the IAC president, Berhane Ras-Work, followed by a mailing of a large information folder on FGM. But not one word was included to discourage medicalization or warn physicians that it is a breech of medical ethics to mutilate a child.

Not until half a year after I wrote to WHO repeatedly, pointing out **their failure and critical omission to oppose medicalization of FGM even though they had opposed medicalization previously,** did WHO add a statement on the subject. Obviously this was much too late, the damage was done as the reaction after the population conference by Egyptian physicians demonstrates. **Had WHO warned against medicalization consistently, backing up their recommendations of Khartoum, the medicalization proposal in Egypt to teach physicians - at government expense - how to do the mutilation, would have never been made.** Health ministries and especially physicians in Africa and the Middle East listen to WHO, which enjoys great prestige and influence around the world.

FINALLY, IT IS IMPORTANT TO BE CLEAR ON WHERE FGM IS PRACTICED AND BY WHOM in order to work for change. This is why, after discovering the existence of FGM, all my efforts were directed to establish these critical facts - that is, the epidemiology of FGM. With so many African refugees recently fleeing their violent continent and trying to settle in Europe, North America as well as Australia, it is important to know where damaging traditions prevail in order to protect the children of the refugees.

The IAC, which was founded in 1984, now has affiliates in 24 African countries and has organized three regional conferences for their members to set priorities and develop policy for the coming years. The most recent one, held in Addis Ababa, also celebrated the IAC's 10th anniversary. They have established and recorded the facts of what is practiced where, and by whom, in each affiliated African country.

Yet recently claims were made in two books that FGM, besides in Africa and in the countries documented in **The HOSKEN REPORT,** is also practiced in Latin American countries and in Pakistan. One of the books even shows a world map, claiming that FGM is practiced in countries all over the world, without providing any facts or documentation. (For a documented geographic overview see the chapter on "Women and Health.")

Until a few years ago it was stated by many international organizations including UNICEF and WHO that FGM is practiced **"in a few remote areas by isolated people"** and that **"the practice is rapidly vanishing."** But to claim now, without providing facts, that FGM is practiced all over the world, is equally damaging especially to the women living in Africa and working to eradicate FGM.

For instance, a world map in the booklet "Female Genital Mutilation" by Nahid Toubia, a Sudanese woman who lives in the US, shows that besides in Africa **and in the countries previously documented,** FGM is practiced in the US (including Alaska), and in Australia, Canada, Brazil, France, India, Israel, Italy, Malaysia, Netherlands, Sweden and United Kingdom. **No sources are cited, no documentation for this information is provided.** The map indicates that less than 1 percent of the population in all the above cited countries practices FGM, **yet this still amounts to many millions of mutilated women. No distinction is made between the populations of these countries and African immigrants from countries where FGM is practiced.** Such undocumented damaging claims may scare people who do not know the facts and result in discrimination against immigrants as well as in tightening of immigration laws.

In the other book, **Cutting the Rose - Female Genital Mutilation,** written by Efua Dorkenoo, a Ghanaian who lives in London, and published by **Minority Rights Publications,** maps show that FGM is practiced in Peru, Brazil, Colombia and Pakistan in addition to sub-Saharan Africa and in the countries documented in **The HOSKEN REPORT.** Again, no documentation is provided, no explanation, and no medical facts. Unfortunately, neither the author nor the publisher answered requests for documentation.

The most reliable way to establish the facts is through midwives and those who attend childbirth, including health workers, at local maternities. I went all over Africa to maternity hospitals, talked to midwives and physicians and assembled all published medical information on the subject. **This information, which had never previously been brought together, was published in my article on the epidemiology of FGM.*** One result was that the WHO seminar was organized, as the excuse that FGM was an isolated practice was no longer creditable. At the seminar I gave a paper on a global review of FGM, including all my research and field work, which was published in the seminar report.

Since then **I have continuously gathered more information and have regularly updated the statistics which are in the chapter on "Women and Health,"** including a factual global overview. FGM statistics in Africa can be tabulated by ethnic group, and it must be updated regularly due to population growth. At present, most existing statistics have been copied from my work, including what is published by WHO. **Unfortunately, what WHO publishes is often outdated, such as their current estimate that 80 million women in Africa are mutilated - the number I documented back in 1982.**

---

*"The Epidemiology of Female Genital Mutilation," **Tropical Doctor,** Royal Society of Medicine, UK, Vol. 8, 1978, pp. 150-156. "Female Circumcision in the World Today: A Global Review," **WHO/EMRO,** Alexandria, Egypt; Vol. 2, 1982, pp. 195-214.

Such claims about the spread of FGM as shown on these recently published maps are very damaging as such information is often picked up and sensationalized by the press, especially since the real facts about FGM are still quite unknown to most of the public. This results in xenophobia and the circulation of all kinds of damaging rumors, and may lead to tightening of immigration laws. Or it may be said that since FGM is so widely practiced there is nothing we can do about it. **Therefore the mutilations should be done "safely" in hospitals,** which was recently proposed in the Netherlands. Fortunately this was stopped due to widespread protests by Dutch women. But as the example of Egypt shows, medicalization will continue to be promoted by the patriarchal medical interests who make money from the operations. **What is really needed is much more support, both technical and financial, for the women in Africa who are fighting to stop FGM; it is in Africa where assistance for eradication needs to be concentrated.**

Immigrants everywhere try to continue their traditions no matter where they go to live. But even moving from a village to a town requires complete change of personal behavior and lifestyle. Moving to another country, no matter what the reason, requires accepting new and different laws and often a new language, quite aside from adapting to a different climate, way of life and environment and learning about different ways to communicate using new technologies. As an immigrant myself, I am quite aware of the necessity to adapt and change: **to learn something new is a challenge and a positive experience that expands your life and is not a hardship, as is often claimed.**

First of all, it is required of all immigrants everywhere to observe the laws of the country where they choose to live. But when it comes to women and children, some immigrant men seem to think the laws which state that all persons have rights of their own do not apply; women are still regarded as the property of men. **Traditions that severely damage women and children are continued with impunity, but the younger generation** must adapt to a very different way of life in order to support themselves. It must be kept in mind that most immigrants, especially those from Africa, represent a small educated elite; the rest of the millions of African refugees of the constant civil wars - mostly women and children - linger in the many refugee camps in Africa, often leading desperate lives.

In the region of Paris where many families from West Africa live, French authorities for a long time ignored the ongoing practice of FGM among immigrants. Though **FGM is criminal child abuse according to French law,** the African immigrants were never warned that to mutilate children is against the law. Only after three little African girls born in France died from excision performed in their parents' homes did the French authorities have to take note. After years of litigation, as the girls' deaths could not be ignored, the French Government belatedly started some information programs for African immigrants. (See **The HOSKEN REPORT** chapter on the "Western World.")

FGM is criminal child abuse according to the laws in most of the world: surely the protection of the lives and health of children must be the foremost priority everywhere. FGM furthermore is classified internationally as human rights violation. (See chapter on "Human Rights.") Many European countries have developed at public expense education programs for African immigrants to protect their children from being mutilated, and special legislation was passed in the UK. In Canada, many positive actions are underway, and the Canadian Health Department recently distributed 2,000 of our **Childbirth Picture Books** in Somali which were translated by Somalian women immigrants living in Canada.

THESE FOUR CRITICAL OBSERVATIONS provide some background for the practice of FGM; they are based on more than 22 years of experience in Africa and research all over the world as well as working with African women to support their concerns. The distribution of the **Childbirth Picture Books** has further contributed to understanding what is needed on the community level to work for change. Many important positive initiatives in Africa are summarized in the chapter on "Actions for Change" in **The HOSKEN REPORT.** But one thing is certain: **it will take much more extensive internationally supported efforts in Africa to eradicate these practices, which has to be done in Africa by the leadership and on the grass roots level.** The IAC has extensive experience and provides a model. Actions for change cannot be done from the outside. They must be led by African women who live in Africa: their courage in performing this difficult and often frustrating task is admirable and deserves all our support. **"I am my sister's keeper"** is what binds us together in solidarity. **As long as some of us are not free, none of us are free.**

WIN NEWS has borne witness to the global revolution by and for women around the world - the most far-reaching social change which is taking place everywhere right now, from the grass roots to the highest level of government and international affairs. The fight to stop FGM and protect our integrity is an essential part of the change we are demanding. Women are speaking up; we are no longer silent. All over the world women are finding that we suffer the same oppression and share the same concerns. But until quite recently our quest for freedom, for a better life and control over our own bodies have been pushed aside by the political power struggles and ambitions of men.

The global women's conferences by the United Nations have given women a unique opportunity to get to know each other first hand, face to face, and as persons in their own right. This has swept away the prejudices women have been taught, each by her own patriarchal family and society. Women everywhere have begun to appreciate the bonds we share, our mutual concerns for our children and for a caring and nurturing environment. From 1975, when the first-ever global women's conference was held in Mexico, to 1995, in Beijing, we have been part - indeed often the instigators - of an overwhelming global revolution of values.

Women all over the world, from women farmers in remote rural areas to women astronauts, from street vendors to prime ministers, have demonstrated their unique abilities, their stamina to survive, their contributions and worth. **We shall no longer serve the ambitions of men, of male rule by violence which has for centuries dominated the world using women and children as pawns.** Through personal contact and communication women everywhere have learned and know that there are other better ways and other goals: human fulfillment cannot be achieved by force and fear.

Women share their revulsion of male violence, of traditional practices that abuse, mutilate and kill girls and women which men use all over the world to impose their control. The fight to stop FGM is the most important example of this global struggle to gain control of our bodies and lives and to set very different goals. Once you see the light, once women realize that there are other better ways and there is hope for change, there is no way we can be forced back. We shall succeed for our children: there is no alternative.

The global patriarchal family system which vests all power in its male head is struggling now to keep up its traditional domination of women and children, using all means including violence, which has recently measurably increased in reaction to women's gains. The status of women around the world has been conclusively researched and recorded in hundreds of books by women since 1975, International Women's Year. **The systematic exploitation of girls and women by economic systems and the abuse of female family members by the global patriarchal family system have been documented** by women's publications and **WIN NEWS.** The record shows that the traditional patriarchal structure of the family functions by denying democratic principles and equal rights.

It is in the family where children are socialized and educated, as Riane Eisler states in her recent editorial for **WIN NEWS** on the Partnership Society:*

> "The link between cruelty and violence in the private sphere of the family and the cruelty and violence of authoritarianism, and other forms of oppression and domination in the political sphere is all too real. . . For the basic fact is that people learn how to behave in their families; they learn what behaviors will be rewarded, punished, or not punished - and thus effectively condoned. And as long as acts of cruelty and violence in people's families are condoned rather than condemned and prosecuted, not only will these continue from generation to generation, but so also will acts of cruelty and violence outside of the family. . ."

The autocratic male dominated family system enforced by violence that prevails around the world and democratic principles of government promoted internationally are bound to collide. A democratic government system requires equality and democracy in the family as the family structure is the backbone of all government.

*Guest editorial by Riane Eisler, **WIN NEWS,** Vol. 19, No. 4, Autumn 1993. See also her books, **The Chalice and the Blade: Our History, Our Future** (ISBN 0-06-250287) and **Sacred Pleasure** (0-06-250293X), both published by Harper & Row, San Francisco.

Women everywhere and ever louder are demanding change. Due to new communication technology women are no longer isolated. Women are getting to know each other across all political and patriarchal boundaries: we are finding that we all share the same concerns. Women are no longer quietly accepting their oppression and their fate to serve the male family head, the male boss, the male general and dictator - with a smile.

Custom and tradition are used everywhere in the world to shore up the collapsing global patriarchal family structure which has always denied women their rights using traditional practices such as violence and FGM as means to that end. The patriarchal family structure compels women to serve men and denies women access to resources and education. Typically, boys are sent to school but girls are kept at home to do household chores.

Wife abuse, "to teach women manners," as the Kenyan Members of Parliament stated recently, is recognized all over Africa and the Middle East as a family tradition. Child marriage, the brideprice (the sale of daughters by the family heads), and polygamy are some of the "customs and traditions" that still flourish today all over Africa. Foot-binding in China and widow burning in India have been abandoned only recently as respected family traditions. But sexual slavery and forced prostitution are flourishing everywhere, especially throughout Southeast Asia to which sex tourism has been recently added.

All this was carefully hidden in the past, but became known worldwide, documented and discussed by women who were no longer isolated in each family from the rest of the world. **The huge barriers between women, from political borders and organizations that teach women to distrust each other, finally were broken when women met face to face.** As reported in **WIN NEWS** it took several years to overcome these damaging walls. By the end of the Decade for Women at the conference in Nairobi, a remarkable consensus developed between women working for shared goals for independence, equality, freedom and human rights.

We need a new world order, we have to change the damaging patriarchal system that holds half the population of the world - women - in bondage to serve the other half - men. We need the contributions of both men and women to make a better, more productive, more satisfying world that is based on equal sharing - on equal contributions by all family members according to their own abilities.

No one has discussed such aspirations, indeed, **a new world order,** better and more persuasively than Riane Eisler in her writings about a new partnership society.

> "Today, as never before in human history, the world stands at a crossroads. On the one side is the well-trodden path of violence and domination - of man over woman, man over man, parent over child, race over race, nation over nation, and man over nature. This is the road leading to a world of totalitarian controls and nuclear or ecological disaster. On the other side lies a very different path: **the road to a world where our basic civil, political, and economic rights - including protection from domination and violence will be respected,** and our natural environment will be protected from man's fabled 'conquest of nature.' This is the road that could take us to a new era of human partnership and peace. In my work I use the terms **domination** and **partnership** in a specific way, to describe two contrasting models of social organization. In **the dominator model,** human differences - beginning with the differences between male and female - are automatically equated with inferiority or superiority, with those deemed 'superior' (men) doing the dominating of those deemed 'inferior' (women). In this model, human rights are, by definition, severely limited, as the whole system is held together by fear and force. . ."

Somalia today is an example where anarchy and violence have taken over and productive social organization has collapsed. The efforts by the Somali women to rid their society of the terrible traditional practice of infibulation which damages every woman and, with it, the whole society, came too late. The violence all over Africa, which has engulfed so many countries of that continent into continuous civil wars and ethnic strife, is in no small way related to family traditions and the treatment of women as inferior and finally as possessions of men.

The traditional patriarchal family model is not compatible with development: this was shown by comparative research, documented by the United Nations on the global status of women and the **Human Development Reports** published annually by the Unted Nations Development Program (UNDP). Most of the poorest countries, according to these statistics, are those where women are most exploited, deprived of property rights, kept in seclusion, illiterate, excised or infibulated and violated by men in their families. The widespread abuse of women was also documented in their testimonies at the 1993 human rights conference in Vienna. (See **WIN NEWS** 19-3, summer '93). **Poverty is not what causes abuse - rather abuse of women is a major cause of poverty and underdevelopment - so all statistics confirm.**

From the economic point of view, it is persuasive to make a major effort to stop the abuse of the female half of society, and especially the mutilation of female children, as the health care costs which are funded by each government are getting ever larger. The cost of work time lost is also paid by the government, which is the largest employer in most countries.

But the loss in human potential, and with it, the loss of the contributions of a large part of the population, cannot be measured only in economic terms. It affects the well being of the whole society. This finally must be recognized internationally by all who are concerned with international development and with population growth, which is directly linked to development.

From an international viewpoint, it is no longer feasible to claim that FGM affects "a few isolated people," as has been done for so long, denying the resulting widespread health damage. **Health and family planning and especially safe motherhood programs will have to acknowledge not only the existence of FGM** but the loss of life and the mounting health costs that the continuation of these practices entails. Instead of treating the eradication of FGM as a separate isolated activity, it is logical as well as far less costly and much more effective **to integrate the prevention of FGM into all family planning, health and safe motherhood programs.** It is obvious to anyone who knows the terrible effects of FGM on childbirth that to seriously work for the reduction of maternal deaths in areas where FGM is practiced **preventive education to stop the mutilations must be integrated into all educational efforts or the whole activity is bound to fail.**

If teaching prevention of FGM is made a part of every health and family planning program, the costs to each one would be very small; prevention would thus be reinforced, accomplishing much more than separate programs. Collaboration in preventive teaching should be organized by all family planning and health programs in African and Middle Eastern countries where FGM is practiced. The teaching experience of the IAC and of AIDoS to prevent FGM certainly can provide viable models on how to proceed.

I have testified repeatedly in Congress before the Foreign Operations Subcommittee of the Appropriations Committee,* which funds USAID, **to support the introduction of preventive education into all USAID population and health programs in Africa** which can be done immediately without additional costs to taxpayers. What is more, the programs are already in place and therefore preventive teaching could start without delay.

The question that must be raised is: **how is it possible that we do nothing while millions of families continue to mutilate their children,** mostly because, contrary to all biological facts, traditional beliefs claim the mutilations are "necessary" for a variety of reasons that seem compelling to the people involved. Most often FGM is a requirement by men for marriage: **the education of African men about the facts of reproduction surely is not beyond the ability of the men in charge of population programs.**

The myths told - and believed - about FGM and the related beliefs in magic and evil spirits have no place in the world today, especially when used for sexual attacks on children. **This is a challenge: surely our ever-expanding communication technology can find ways to teach all people the basic facts about their own bodies and reproduction** - even if they cannot read - and that is what is needed first of all. That is why I developed the **Childbirth Picture Book** as soon as I returned from the Khartoum seminar, based on the recommendations on education. (See Appendix, **Childbirth Picture Book Program.**)

---

* Testimonies of 1993, 1994 and 1995 are available from **WIN NEWS.**

Today, the greatest danger is posed by the medicalization of FGM, which is growing throughout Africa as cited above. Medicalization was already discussed in 1979 at the Khartoum seminar when the Sudanese physicians, backed by the WHO representative from Geneva, Dr. Bannerman, demanded that the recommendations - which have guided all actions in Africa every since - be formulated to include medicalization as an option. After a day-long acrimonious debate this option was finally dropped due to the adamant opposition of Dr. Bertha Johnson, a psychiatrist from Nigeria, the ranking woman physician at the seminar, and the opposition by the secretary of the conference, Dr. Baasher of the WHO regional office in Alexandria.

But of course this has not stopped physicians all over Africa and other parts of the world from making money by mutilating female children, supported by African politicians who still demand FGM but prefer medicalization for their own families.

The failure of organized medical and health professionals around the world to oppose this outrageous abuse and criminal violation of medical ethics is responsible for the introduction of FGM into medical practice around the world. Where are the physicians to openly attack such medical malpractice? Where are the leaders of the health professions? Why do they not speak for women's integrity and human rights?

The experience on the grass roots level with the Childbirth Picture Books is convincing: there are hundreds of community groups all over Africa, ready, willing and eager to teach prevention and stop FGM in their own local communities; indeed they are already doing it and need to be strengthened. With support - including technical help and training, teaching materials and salaries for hiring local help - they could reach many more people. As the letters asking for Childbirth Picture Books from so many local groups and people all over Africa confirm, this grass roots movement has enormous potential - especially since men are also involved.

The Peace Corps provides another model - for instance, funding a domestic peace corps in African countries could greatly help local development. Young people in urban areas who want to go on to higher education in return for scholarships would go to rural areas to teach for a year or two about basic health, prevention of FGM, literacy, and whatever local people need. (See Appendix.) The IAC, with 11 years of field experience and affiliates all over Africa, should not only be consulted but funded in such a way that they are able to carry out what they know needs to be done to effectively deal with prevention. And prevention would make medicalization redundant and unnecessary.

Many years ago when I first learned the facts about FGM, like many other women I was unwilling to face the truth. Nothing in my experience and life in Europe and the US or in my many travels all over the world had prepared me for such revelations; they forced me to re-think and re-examine everything I had believed and I had learned. But from all my travels in Africa and my many conversations with women from all different countries and backgrounds, what the midwives in the city hospital in Bamako told me, after describing the problems of FGM and women in their society, has stayed with me ever since: change cannot be partial to be effective; everything must change; our whole society must be reorganized until women take their rightful place.

We must take our rightful place everywhere in the world. No one will give it to us, least of all those who enjoy all the privileges of their domination and control. In the worldwide revolution by women to gain control over their own bodies and lives, the eradication of genital mutilations is an imperative. It is both a symbol as well as a cornerstone. In the battle for freedom of choice, the issue of female genital mutilation is a fundamental and pivotal political concern.

HEALTH FACTS AND OVERVIEW

This summary of the health facts of female genital mutilation (FGM) should be read first. It gives essential background information for the rest of this book. Detailed documentation is provided in **The HOSKEN REPORT - Genital and Sexual Mutilation of Females,** especially in the country case histories, where field investigations in Africa and research are brought together. **The HOSKEN REPORT** documents that female genital mutilation is a major public health problem that has damaged the health and lives of more than 120 million girls and women in continental Africa, and millions more are mutilated every year. Since the health of so many women and girls is seriously injured by FGM, national development is damaged in more than 26 countries in a vast area from the Red Sea in the east to the Atlantic coast of West Africa. The mutilations are also practiced in the southern part of the Arab Peninsula and in a less damaging form by some Moslem groups in Malaysia and Indonesia.

Recently, it has been found that African and Middle Eastern immigrants to Europe, North America and Australia, mostly refugees, continue to practice these mutilations on their children, no matter where they go to live, though these operations are prohibited by local child-abuse laws. Information and education programs have been organized in many countries to stop them.

The HOSKEN REPORT, which provides the research for this book, was first published in 1979 by **WIN NEWS.** The fourth revised and updated edition came out in January 1994. The report established for the first time the epidemiology as well as the history of FGM, and documents how widespread these mutilations are, which was hidden for 2,000 years. However, though the facts are now known, all development, health and population programs working in the affected countries continue to ignore the torturous and often life-threatening damage done to girls and women. (See chapter on "Politics" of **The HOSKEN REPORT.**) **The current $450 million annual budget for population by the US Agency for International Development (USAID) includes nothing for prevention of FGM.**

In the quarterly journal of Women's International Network - **WIN NEWS,** [1] which I began publishing in 1975, new information on FGM is reported in every issue. **WIN NEWS** also continuously reports on our **grass roots initiative** of **distributing our Childbirth Picture Books (CBPB)** [2] **with their Additions to Prevent Excision and Infibulation** to local community health groups all over Africa and the Middle East. These educational materials, produced in many languages, teach with pictures the biological facts of reproduction, regardless of language or literacy. The Additions show the health problems resulting from the mutilations, especially in childbirth, to demystify the damaging traditional beliefs. The **CBPBs** are well understood, according to hundreds of letters we receive from recipients.

This book reports what women from all over Africa say and think about FGM. But it is also a fact that these traditional practices do great damage to the economy of each society and country as is documented in the country case studies of **The HOSKEN REPORT.** (See cost analysis below.) But the **terrible suffering and severe psychological trauma** that FGM imposes on female children and women at an early age and throughout their lives can never be measured. They are a social burden of sexual violence imposed by the traditional patriarchal system on those least able to protect themselves. To defend such practices on cultural grounds is a distortion of the meaning of culture. Recently it has also been documented that FGM contributes to the spread of HIV/AIDS, which is increasing more rapidly among women in sub-Saharan Africa than anywhere, and is therefore infecting more and more children.

Little girls who are subjected to these mutilations, often only a few weeks or years old, cannot make any decisions on their own and do not know what is done to them. They and their mothers have no choice and are not only **ignorant of the health dangers involved and the lifelong suffering the operations cause, but they are also unaware of the most basic reproductive facts and that FGM is not practiced in most of the world.** Many women believe that these mutilations are necessary to have children. Different myths are told by different ethnic groups why girls must undergo FGM, and girls are treated as outcasts by their families if they refuse. The real reason why FGM continues is that African men refuse to marry women who are not operated.

Those of us who know the truth **must take responsibility for making information about reproduction and sexuality known and available everywhere**, especially to the victims of these damaging practices so their daughters will be spared. In our age of electronic communication where information can instantly reach all over the world, why are the most basic facts about human biology and reproduction still concealed?

In Africa, the term "female circumcision" is still popular, though medically incorrect. It is used for a variety of mutilating genital operations by local traditional operators, mostly women but also men in some countries, who are well paid for their services. At the 1990 conference in Addis Ababa by the **Inter-African Committee on Traditional Practices Affecting the Health of Women and Children (IAC),**[3] the delegations from more than 20 African countries unanimously stated that **female genital mutilation** is the term that should be used internationally. The World Health Organization (WHO), UNICEF and all other international agencies concerned with health have done so since.

From a biological and health view the operations on girls are not a counterpart to male circumcision - though both operations are often done as puberty rites. What is done to girls has a different purpose and result: a healthy and most sensitive organ of a woman's body is amputated. **The genital mutilations performed on girls are quite different from the operation on boys. FGM is the equivalent of the amputation of part or all of the penis** - with very similar physical and sexual results (see comparison below).

For Moslems, the removal of the foreskin of boys is a religious requirement demanded by the Koran. It is also a requirement for "manhood" throughout tribal Africa. But there is no requirement for a female operation anywhere in the Koran as Moslem religious authorities have confirmed. Nevertheless, some local Moslem sheiks and leaders preach that "female circumcision is a religious requirement." Women, most of whom can neither read nor write, have no choice but to accept what these men of religion claim. But FGM is practiced by African followers of all religions including Christians - Catholics, Protestants, Copts - and is tolerated by most male religious leaders.

Since some African and Arab traditionalists still object to calling these female genital operations a mutilation, the definition of the word should be examined. According to Webster, to mutilate (from "mutilus" - maimed) means "to cripple, to injure, to damage, or otherwise make imperfect, especially by removing an essential part or parts." **The term mutilation quite correctly describes what is done by the operations** - which remove the most sensitive organ of the female body, without medical indication.

The female genitalia that are created "perfect" are deliberately crippled and altered according to custom. It is men who determine what becomes a custom and finally a tradition in each society. The objective, which is quite openly stated by African and Middle Eastern men, is to deprive women of sexual pleasure and to keep women under male control. In Moslem countries, women are told that they are unable to control their sexuality; therefore they must be excised. In different ethnic groups, the genital operations take different forms and are performed on girls of different ages, with a variety of different reasons given (see below). The purpose and medical results, however, are the same.

Physicians so far have failed to organize international actions on medical grounds to stop FGM, though the facts are known everywhere. All over the world men have formed organizations to stop health abuses of every kind, and professional men are involved in many health-related international initiatives. **Why is there no organization of medical men against FGM,** to stop health practitioners and physicians from doing the mutilations and to stop men from having their daughters mutilated? Men in power must be told by international leaders of the medical profession and in turn by those in the health leadership in each African country that these mutilations are unacceptable. WHO has representatives in all African countries, but these WHO officials have been mute.

In Africa and the Middle East, fathers arrange the marriages of their daughters and they collect the bride-price: therefore they see to it that their **daughters are mutilated - as FGM is a marriage requirement;** the money and gifts (the "brideprice") a fathers gets for his daughter is considerable, so the girls are often sold very young. Since women have no alternative but marriage, the mutilations continue. African men claim the operations are a "women's affair," refusing to take responsibility. But if men rejected marriage with mutilated women, the practice would stop immediately. **Where is the leadership of men?**

DEFINITIONS OF THE OPERATIONS

Three kinds of operations are described in the medical literature. These definitions by gynecologists are derived from observations and case histories, that is, after the fact, rather than by the operators who have no knowledge of anatomy. All the operations are performed without anesthetic, often on struggling children held down by force, frequently on the ground under highly septic conditions, using a variety of tools. These definitions are summarized from descriptions given throughout the medical literature.

1. **Sunna Circumcision (Sunna means "tradition" in Arabic)**
   Removal of the prepuce and the tip of the clitoris (mildest form). This delicate operation cannot be performed by traditional operators, given the lack of anatomical knowledge of the operators, the crude tools used and the environmental conditions (operations are done on the ground, in dark huts, under trees, etc.).

2. **Excision/Clitoridectomy**
   Removal of the clitoris and often adjacent parts including the labia minora and all exterior genitalia. In some areas, additional cuts into the vagina are added, for instance, in Kenya or Sierra Leone, "to make childbirth easier"; the opposite is true. Excision is the most frequent operation; damage depends on the local practices.

3. **Infibulation (Pharaonic Circumcision)**
   After the removal of the clitoris and labia minora as well as parts of the labia majora, the two sides of the vulva are closed over the vagina. This is done by fastening together the bleeding sides of the labia majora with thorns or catgut or some sticky paste. A small opening is created by inserting a splinter of wood to allow for elimination of urine and later menstrual blood. The legs of the child are then tied together, immobilizing her for several weeks or until the wound is healed, closing the opening to the vagina.

The mortality of girls and women due to these operations is high, but no records are kept. Primary fatalities are not recorded; death in childbirth, due to obstructed labor caused by the mutilations, is never related to genital operations.

Excision/clitoridectomy in Africa is popularly called "female circumcision" and describes all kinds of genital operations, the extent of which can only be determined by gynecological examination. The damage done, or the severity of the operation, depends on local customs, on the operator's skill and on the tools used. Traditionally, special knives are used, although sharp stones or glass were also used in the past, and recently, razor blades. The more traditional the ethnic group, the more drastic the operation; that is, the more flesh is removed.

Old women, traditional birth attendants who are sometimes called midwives though they have no health training, perform the operations in most of Africa and the Middle East. **In some areas, excision is an inherited trade and special "excisors" go from village to village.** Sometimes male operators are involved; for instance, barbers in northern Nigeria and Egypt do the operations. Physicians now perform the operations on the children of the wealthy for a fee, in Sudan, Nigeria, Egypt, Kenya and Somalia, and no doubt in many other countries. Hospitals are also doing them for a fee - for instance, all over Kenya, in Mali and elsewhere. African health personnel, trained by international health and population programs that have access to imported antibiotics, make extra money by doing them, without objection by the international sponsors. **The medicalization of FGM is rapidly increasing, but WHO has utterly failed to stop this.**
Infibulation is known as "Pharaonic Circumcision" because it always has been practiced in Upper Egypt and was known to the ancient Egyptians. The term "infibulation" goes back to the Romans. **Fibula means clasp or pin in Latin.** A fibula was used to hold together the toga, the loose garment worn by Roman men. To prevent sexual intercourse, the Romans fastened a fibula through the large lips of women and a ring or fibula through the foreskin of men - usually slaves.[4] Infibulated female slaves from Upper Egypt and Sudan fetched a higher price on the slave markets of Cairo up to the 19th century, as childbearing hampers their work.

Infibulation may also occur spontaneously by adherence of the wounded sides of the labia, especially where extensive excision operations are performed, such as in Mali, Burkina Faso and parts of Senegal.

The objective of infibulation is to make sexual intercourse impossible. At present, infibulation is practiced as a rule chiefly by Moslems, according to all available sources, because of **the importance Moslems attach to virginity. Infibulation is performed to guarantee that a bride is intact - the smaller her opening, the higher the brideprice.** A girl is often inspected by the female relatives of the husband-to-be before the brideprice is paid, for instance in Somalia.

Women who are infibulated have to be cut open to allow penetration - and more cuts are needed for delivery of a child. Wives, traditionally, are re-infibulated in Sudan and Somalia after the baby is born; when the child is weaned, they are opened again for intercourse. During her reproductive life, a woman used to go through this process with each child, and in some areas it still continues today. The decision rests with the husband, who has several wives. For instance, the Somali men who came to the Benadir Hospital - the largest hospital for women and children in Mogadishu - demanded that their wives be re-infibulated after delivery, so the head nurse told me. And the same request was made by Somali refugees in Canada after women delivered.

In Sudan, it has been reported that **women often demand re-infibulation** after delivery, claiming this makes intercourse more pleasurable for the husband. A woman must please sexually, or she is divorced, which means loss of her children, loss of all economic support and disgrace for her and her family. It has also been the custom for men to have their wives re-infibulated when they leave home for extended periods of time.

In West Africa, where infibulation is less often done by sewing or other fastening devices, the same results are achieved by tying the legs of the girl together in a crossed position after the operation. After a radical excision operation the scars may completely obliterate the opening to the vagina, as is reported in the medical literature; hospitals report girls being brought in bloated from retention of urine or menstrual blood.

On a visit to Ouagadougou, Burkina Faso, in 1977, while I was in the maternity hospital, a woman in labor with her first child arrived: she could not deliver as she was almost completely closed. There was nothing left at all of her external genitalia. She had evidently conceived through a tiny opening - as is also reported in the medical literature.

Excisions and infibulations are usually performed on the ground, under septic conditions, with the same knife or tool used on all the girls of a group operation. In cases of fatalities, most often the result of cutting a blood vessel, neither the operator nor the operation is ever blamed, even if the girl dies. The conditions under which the mutilations are done provide the opportunity for the transmission of HIV/AIDS; there are more cases of AIDS reported in sub-Saharan Africa especially of women than anywhere in the world.

The locations for the operations vary: under a special tree outside the village, in a designated wood or bush, inside huts, in the backyard, sometimes furtively at dawn. In Sudan, the operation takes place in the home or a walled yard in the presence of many women. Men may not attend the noisy "celebration," though young boys do. In many ethnic groups in Central and West Africa, men participate in the village celebrations but are not allowed to be present at the cutting. Everywhere fathers pay the fees for the operations. The male village elders in sub-Saharan Africa decide when the operations are to be done, while the fathers present their daughters.

The health sector worldwide is controlled by men, internationally as well as in each country. WHO headquarters in Geneva issued in June of 1982 a position statement: **"Female circumcision is a traditional practice which can have serious health consequences and is of concern to the World Health Organization. WHO has consistently and unequivocally advised that female circumcision should not be practiced by any health professionals in any settings - including hospitals or other health establishments."** Though WHO has representatives in all African countries they have failed to support this statement with any action. However, the IAC, with affiliates in more than 24 African countries, has continuously campaigned against medicalization.

Many trained health workers and physicians in Africa perform the mutilations to make money. As I testified repeatedly since 1980 in Congress before the Foreign Operations Subcommittee of the Appropriations Committee, none of the USAID-funded health and population programs in Africa have introduced preventive measures nor do they stop their trained African employees from doing the operations for extra income.

Traditionally the operations are performed at various ages, from newborn babies (for example, in Ethiopia and among the Yoruba in Nigeria) to girls in puberty. The Masai in Kenya and Tanzania are said to perform the operations on the wedding night. In Mali, the midwives in the Gabriel Toure Hospital in Bamako state that in some ethnic groups a woman is excised after her first child in order to keep her faithful to her husband, who has several wives.

In most of sub-Saharan Africa the operations traditionally were performed as a puberty or coming-of-age rite on girls 12 to 15 years old or just before menstruation. **Recently, the age at which excisions are performed has lowered** in the towns, and also in some rural areas where education has spread. The procedure has been stripped of all "traditions"- but the cutting continues. (See **The HOSKEN REPORT:** Kenya.)

Infibulation was traditionally practiced on children ages 6 to 9, and has recently been performed on girls as young as 3 years old in urban areas, for instance, in Sudan or Somalia. Awa Thiam in **Parole aux Negresses,** [5] tells the story of a young woman from Mali who only discovered that she was infibulated when she was to be married. She had no memory of the operation and was kept in ignorance about her condition until her father had arranged her marriage.

Many of the traditional ceremonies surrounding the operations have been greatly simplified or quite abandoned under the impact of modernization, especially in urban areas. However, the mutilations continue to be performed on ever younger children, as parents are afraid their daughters, once they learn what is in store for them, will refuse. Girls living in towns are sometimes brought back to their villages and forcibly subjected to FGM. The grandmothers and older women of the family see to it that all the girls are operated on. However, the decisions in each family are made by men, who demand that all girls are "done." **Men pay for the operations, negotiate the marriage and take the bride-price.** In many ethnic groups, girls who are not mutilated are considered unfit for marriage. That means the father cannot collect the bride-price, therefore, he has his daughters mutilated. In turn, a father will not pay for a bride for his son nor will a man buy a wife who is not excised. Thus, **the operations continue, due to male demands.** Marriage is obligatory for all throughout Africa and the Middle East, and it is strongly advocated by the Koran.

The operations are now performed in the modern health sector of many African cities, for instance, in Mali, Somalia, Nigeria, Sudan, Egypt, Kenya, and more. The operation may be done in a hospital, an infirmary or at the private office of a physician, depending on what the father is willing to pay. If the daughter dies from the operation, the father loses the bride-price. Hence there is an incentive is to use modern health care - that is, imported tools, antibiotics and surgical techniques. For instance, physicians in Sudan and Egypt do the mutilations quite routinely in their offices.

Many village girls who have learned about the pain of the operation try to run away - the only place to go is to the nearest town or the capital. Since they have no skills and are illiterate, the only way they can survive and earn a living is through prostitution. African towns and cities are overflowing with prostitutes - many of them infected with HIV/ AIDS.

Almost every family in West Africa has lost at least one daughter due to FGM - which is one reason why the mutilations are now practiced on ever younger children, so the midwives in the Gabriel Toure Hospital in Bamako told me. The hospital now has excisors right on the premises to mutilate the newborn babies; if anything goes wrong there is help immediately available, so the midwives say.

In recent years, more and more African refugees fleeing to **Europe** and **North America** have brought their customs with them. In most European countries, where health services are paid for by their governments, health ministries alerted all hospitals and physicians that these mutilations are prohibited as criminal child abuse. In Great Britain, special legislation was passed in 1985 after it was reported that a physician had performed the operation in his office in London on the wife of a wealthy African who demanded this as "cure against her infertility."

In **France,** where large numbers of immigrants from West Africa live and work around Paris, **the French Government had to take action** after several little girls born to Malian immigrants died as a result of the mutilation. After ignoring FGM for many years, the matter is now in the criminal courts. Though an information campaign was belatedly started, more cases continuously come to light.

In **Canada,** which recently had a large influx of Somalian refugees (all women in Somalia are infibulated), the College of Physicians and Surgeons of Ontario warned all their members against performing the mutilations and provided specific information how to take care of infibulated women.[6] The Health Ministry also distributed 2,000 of our **Childbirth Picture Books** translated into Somali with the Additions to Prevent Infibulation.

By contrast, in the **Netherlands,** which also accepted many Somalian refugees, physicians in the summer of 1992 discussed the legalization of FGM as a medical procedure done in hospitals, paid for by the government. Under the pretext that immigrants cannot be "robbed of their traditions," medical personnel proposed to operate on the small daughters of immigrants. After many protests by women the government finally declared that they opposed the operations and are teaching immigrants why they are prohibited.

FGM was repeatedly discussed by the press in **Australia**, but no one has been able to document any cases of mutilations actually performed there. Legal authorities have recently taken note, as reported in **WIN NEWS,** which has a continuing section on all developments regarding the spread of FGM.

The facts regarding FGM done by immigrants on their daughters in the **United States** have never been documented though no doubt the mutilations are practiced. The physician/ patient privacy rules protect the practice, and since health care is not paid for by the government, physicians can do whatever they want or get paid for.[7] At this writing, not a single case of FGM done in the US has been medically documented.

However, in 1980, a Sunday newspaper supplement, **The National Black Monitor,** advocated the introduction of FGM into the African-American community. The supplement was distributed to local community papers all over the country, published by a consortium of publishers of African-American papers - all men. One of the editorials urged importing "the beneficial African custom of FGM as a social safeguard" to prevent "teen sex and parenthood" and to "control the sexual waywardness in girls." These self-appointed male leaders of African-American communities suggested "hygienic experimentation with female circumcision" to introduce the mutilation in the US! After a letter writing campaign organized by **WIN NEWS,** the **Black Monitor** editors had to explain the truth about FGM and apologize to women.

FGM has been cited as **a human rights violation** in the **Country Reports on Human Rights Practices,** issued every year by the Department of State (see **WIN NEWS** Spring issues), as well as by the United Nations Commission on Human Rights. In the spring of 1991, a seminar on "Traditional Practices Affecting the Health of Women and Children" was held in Burkina Faso, sponsored by the United Nations Center for Human Rights. Fifteen countries participated, most of them from West Africa. FGM was the main topic of the agenda. [8] The participation of so many West African governments in this conference is remarkable, considering that only a few years earlier the subject of FGM could not be discussed in any meeting in Africa.

Until the WHO seminar in Khartoum in 1979, African and Middle Eastern leaders silenced every attempt to discuss FGM. Indeed, President Kenyatta made FGM a requirement among his ethnic group, the Kikuyu, and his followers in Kenya; he also influenced the leaders all over Africa. It was therefore especially important that his successor, President Daniel arap Moi, categorically prohibited FGM throughout Kenya since1982.

But though education and information programs have been initiated in many countries, most under the guidance of the IAC and some with governmental support - in Burkina Faso, for instance, positive results have been difficult to document. One reason is that far too few resources are supporting these campaigns. Also, all health care and especially maternity services have been drastically cut back due to the World Bank "Austerity and Structural Adjustment" rules that have further devastated the ailing African economies. What is more, internationally funded population and health programs are still ignoring FGM, thus doing terrible damage to women.

DAMAGE TO HEALTH

The health facts given here are summarized from the medical literature and from direct information from midwives and physicians in Africa.

The most important clinical study is a survey of 4,024 women, published in the Sudan Medical Journal, by Dr. Ahmed Abu-El Futuh Shandall. [9] This study of actual case histories observed by the author in the Khartoum Hospital over a period of many years also lists the types of operations encountered and tabulates the statistics of health problems resulting from genital operations. Dr. Shandall goes beyond citing the medical facts and health statistics and makes important suggestions for abolishing the mutilations.

A comprehensive summary of the medical literature concerning damage to physical health resulting from infibulation (Pharaonic circumcision) was edited by Dr. R. Cook when he worked in the Eastern Mediterranean Regional Office of WHO. [10] This paper covers medical publications on female genital operations from 1931 to 1976, providing an overview of the realities of the health problems of women subjected to these procedures.

In the British medical journal **Tropical Doctor**, Dr. J. A. Verzin published an article, **"Sequelae of Female Circumcision,"** [11] which provides a thorough survey of the immediate and long-range health problems resulting from genital mutilation from evidence encountered in medical practice.

In the above-named publications and in other medical literature on FGM the following health problems are recorded:

●   **Immediate Results:** Primary fatalities resulting from hemorrhage (uncontrolled bleeding); shock due to blood loss and pain (no anesthetic is given); septicemia (blood poisoning); infections of the wound, including tetanus, which is fatal; retention of urine immediately following the operation due to occlusion or because of pain when urinating; trauma (injury) to adjacent tissues - the rectum, the urethra; failure of the wound to heal and spreading of the infections as tools are never sterilized.

In some areas, especially in West Africa, the operators throw dirt on the wound to stop the bleeding; ashes and pulverized animal feces are also used, resulting in fatal infections. Many traditional treatments applied to the wounds increase the damage and danger of the operations. Excision by cauterization (burning) is also reported in the literature, resulting in extensive infections and scars.

●   **Long-range Results:** Urinary problems due to chronic infection, which also may lead to infertility; difficulty in passing urine as well as menstrual blood and painful menstruation; malformations, including cysts. Keloid formation (hardening of the scars) is especially prevalent among Negroid peoples causing obstructed labor which may result in death in childbirth.

Many coital difficulties are reported, especially where infibulation is practiced. Often the bride must be cut open before penetration can take place, which causes injury and more infections. Excision can also result in an almost complete closing of the vagina by adherence of the excision wound, which is reported in West Africa and elsewhere in areas where excision is extreme.

Lack of orgasm is reported where studies on this subject were made. Women in many societies are not aware that intercourse can be pleasurable for them. Painful coitus is the most frequent result of the operations, and sexual intercourse recalls the pain of the mutilation. Women are required to submit to intercourse upon the husband's requests at any time.

There are many difficulties in childbirth due to the excision scars which prevent dilation - tears, hemorrhage and infections often result. Delay in labor and prolonged second-stage labor as well as uterine inertia are reported; obstructed labor is a frequent result; sometimes brain damage or death of the baby due to lack of oxygen occurs, especially with the first child. The highest maternal and infant mortality rates in the world are recorded in the regions where genital mutilation is practiced. But the "Safe Motherhood" campaigns organized since 1987 by WHO , the World Bank and other governmental and private agencies are deliberately ignoring FGM - despite the African statistics on FGM and despite the IAC and their affiliates who have made the facts known.

In the case of infibulation, unassisted childbirth is impossible; if there is no one to cut the infibulation huge tears result: both mother and baby often die. The formation of vesico/vaginal (or recto/vaginal) fistulae (rupturing of the vaginal wall) are frequent due to obstructed labor, causing incontinence. This makes the women outcasts of their families and communities as they are continuously dribbling urine and feces. The Kenyatta Hospital in Nairobi, for instance, always has a waiting list of hundreds of women for fistula operations, which are difficult procedures that often fail.

Women with fistulae can be found in most African hospitals in all areas where genital mutilation is practiced, though only a few hospitals can perform these difficult operations which require special aftercare for several weeks. In Addis Ababa, a unique privately-organized Fistula Clinic, run by a husband and wife physician team from Australia and New Zealand, has the highest success rate and is teaching doctors how to do these difficult operations. (See **The HOSKEN REPORT**: Ethiopia.)

● **Psychological Results and Sex Trauma:** The effects of the extreme pain and shock of the operations, as well as the prolonged suffering afterward, have never been conclusively investigated. Only one study exists at present, by Dr. T. A. Baasher, which analyzes the responses of 70 women to a questionnaire about their opinions concerning circumcision.[12] But this study does not deal with the lifelong psychological effects on the mental health of mutilated women. **The permanent psychological damage of this torture to which often very young girls are subjected by their own families, those they love and trust, has been quite ignored.**

The debilitating pain of menstruation (as a result of the operation), the agony of the first intercourse, especially for the infibulated, the prolonged suffering in childbirth, no doubt create deep psychological wounds as well as physical ones. No clinical investigation exists on the subject. At the present time, most women and young girls who are subjected to these operations in Africa are unaware that any alternatives exist or that these mutilations are not practiced in most of the world. Up to 80 percent of the women in rural areas of many African countries where FGM continues to be practiced are still illiterate.

The effects of sexual castration (which these operations actually are) on the personality development of a girl have also been quite ignored. Yet it is clear that the permanent deprivation of a human being's most powerful instinct has deeply depressing psychological results, especially since in Africa and the Middle East a woman's chief purpose in life is to serve the sexual satisfaction of her husband and to bear "his" children.

Those concerned with health in Africa have failed to investigate the psychological results of FGM on children and women and have ignored the health damage by the pervasive rape and sexual violence that is practiced by African men under the label of "cultural practices." The medical literature reports occasionally on the physical damage sustained by girls and young women - their genitalia torn due to the brutal sexual attacks by men, often their husbands, for instance, in Ethiopia, where child marriage is widely practiced. In every hospital maternity ward information is available on severely injured girls due to sexual violence, but no one cares. The psychological results are largely ignored in the medical literature. Suicides by desperate young women, unable to cope with the sexual ordeals to which they are subjected by their husbands as well as the torture of repeated childbirth, are reported, for instance, in Burkina Faso.

Genital mutilation can only be understood in the context of the psychological climate created by the pervasive male domination and sexual violence that form the unseen background of African and Middle Eastern family life. While women in the West have only recently started to speak about male family violence, it is still a mute subject in Africa. For instance, a few years ago, when new family legislation was discussed in Kenya, African Parliamentarians insisted that wife abuse, as a hallowed African tradition, be confirmed by law as the right of every African man.

The physical injuries that can be seen in hospitals are only the tip of the iceberg. The apathy and fatalism that can be observed among many African and Middle Eastern women in rural areas are their psychological defenses against the traditional sexual violence and trauma they suffer from men of their own families from which they are unable to escape.

The feudal social order of communities, which still prevails in most rural areas, is characterized by group behavior that does not recognize individual responsibility by men for violence against women. Decisions are made by the male elders. The bride-price, which is still the rule in almost all African ethnic groups as well as in the Middle East, is nothing more than a price negotiated between men for the sale of women. If a woman does not produce offspring in a given time, she is returned and the bride-price has to be returned . Polygamy is practiced throughout Africa and the Middle East, though most men are unable to support even one wife and her children. Polygamy also contributes to the spread of AIDS. Women have no rights, but are held responsible for all food production.

Traditionally, hunting and warfare were the predominant occupations of African men, and the latter continues up to the present. **No other area in the world has as many civil wars and continuous bloody conflicts** as recently reported, for instance, in Liberia, Somalia, Sudan, Ethiopia, Mozambique, Uganda, Rwanda, Angola, Nigeria, South Africa, and more - quite aside from constant local ethnic conflicts not reported by the international press. No other continent has as many refugees: women and children are, predictably, the vast majority of the victims of this constant warfare and violence by men.

These violent traditional practices are never discussed by anthropologists, most of whom praise "culture and tradition" no matter how damaging to women and children - and despite the fact that many traditional practices are recognized as human rights violations by the United Nations. **The horrendous reality of the famine and brutal civil and tribal warfare by men** in Somalia was shown daily on television for many months. But no one commented that the Somali men and boys with guns were well fed and healthy, while the women and children were starving and dying. If African society is to survive and flourish on this huge, beautiful and richly endowed continent, the attitudes and customs of men must change.

While the recurring African droughts can be dealt with by temporary organized efforts from outside, **the rapidly declining agricultural production all over Africa requires a re-orientation of customs and traditions by men. Change in male behavior has to start within each family where boys learn violence from their fathers.** The equality and dignity of women and children who are the productive members of African society must be recognized.

Women produce most of the food that African families need to survive; their contributions must be officially recognized. Women have earned the right to participate in all governments and decisions as equals if democracy means anything at all. Men must share in food production rather than only growing cash crops.

REASONS GIVEN

Many colorful myths are related all over Africa as reasons for the mutilations. Though all the myths are still believed by the ethnic groups involved especially in the rural areas, many of the reasons are contradictory and none are compatible with biological facts.

Most Africans who practice these mutilations believe that these customs are decreed by their ancestors or their religion. But the decisive factor is that men refuse to marry women who are not excised. Since marriage is still the only career for a woman in most of Africa and the Middle East, the operations continue.

"No proper Kikuyu will marry a girl who has not been circumcised" is the frequently cited statement by Jomo Kenyatta, the revered leader of Kenya. In his book, which was written in the 1930's but continues to be published and is sold in bookstores in Nairobi to tourists this statement is also included. [13] The book explains the customs of the Kikuyu, the dominant population group of Kenya, who still control Kenya's political life. As president of Kenya for life, Kenyatta had great influence on Africans well beyond the borders of Kenya, and **this much quoted pronouncement is responsible for the mutilation of millions of helpless little girls and untold suffering and deaths all over Africa.**

Excision, cutting out the most sensitive organ of a woman's body, extinguishes sexual sensitivity and response to touch. That this is recognized in Africa and the Middle East is confirmed by **the reasons most frequently given for the operations: "to keep moral behavior of women in society" and "to assure the faithfulness of women to their husbands,"** who usually have several wives. In sub-Saharan Africa the operation traditionally is performed as a puberty rite; it is claimed that a woman can be accepted into adult society and get married only after she is excised.

In Sudan and the Middle East and in Moslem societies, it is said that **a woman is incapable of controlling her sexuality** - hence she must be excised and infibulated, or she will disgrace her family. Infibulation is traditionally performed on much younger children than excision or long before puberty. A girl who is not mutilated is risking her and her family's status in society and is considered to be a prostitute. Infibulation is practiced mostly in devout Moslem areas to visibly guarantee chastity. The honor of the patriarchal family is involved, hence she has no choice. Women are objects of trade between men, who have up to four wives. Yet this does not prevent frequent divorces. After divorce a woman is re-infibulated by her family and sold again to another man. Infibulation, it is believed, assures the husband that the children of the woman he purchased are his own. (See **The HOSKEN REPORT**: Somalia.)

In most ethnic groups excision traditionally was, and is, a coming-of-age rite, performed at puberty on girls 12 to 14 years old or just before menstruation and marriage. In a few ethnic groups the operation is done after marriage, so some reports state. Traditionally, groups of girls are excised together in a secluded location outside the village under a special tree or in a secret bush that no one is allowed to enter (see **The HOSKEN REPORT**: Sierra Leone). Excision is a marriage requirement, no man will pay bride-price for a girl who is not mutilated. The village chief determines the day and time for the excision procedure - after consulting the "spirits." Traditionally, the girls are kept in seclusion for several weeks or longer after the operation and are instructed in the "duties" of a wife. **If a girl dies, it is blamed on her, never on the operator or the mutilation, or it is said that the ritual was not properly performed according to the rules.**

Initiations involving excision and clitoridectomy are also practiced by Christian converts of all denominations. In the past, some of the Protestant missionaries, such as the Scottish Church Missionary Society in Kenya in the 1920's, strongly opposed these operations, but little or nothing is said against them now. **The Roman Catholics Church officially condoned genital mutilation of the children of their converts,** because the Catholic community would diminish, the Catholic leaders said, since men refused to marry girls who were not excised (see **The HOSKEN REPORT**: History). There are more mutilated Catholic women all over Africa than in those of other Christian religions.

Because the biological facts about reproduction are unknown, **it is widely believed that a woman who is not excised is unable to have children. Excision is also perceived as a method to increase fertility.** Since the status of women in African society depends on having many children, especially sons, infertility is truly a tragedy for an African woman.

In Mali, Burkina Faso and all over West Africa, the people claim that the clitoris connotes maleness while the prepuce of the penis represents femaleness. Hence, both have to be removed before a person can be accepted as an adult in his/her sex and society. In Burkina Faso and much of Francophone Africa, **the clitoris is viewed as a dangerous organ** that will kill the baby during childbirth and therefore must be removed. Another widely told myth is that the clitoris will damage the husband's genitalia during intercourse and injure him or make him infertile. The Bambara in West Africa claim the clitoris is the equivalent of the penis and must be removed before childbearing is possible.

In Ethiopia and Sudan, it is said that **a girl who is not operated will run wild and disgrace her family. The operation needs to be done to "calm" a girl** and make her submissive. **In Egypt, aesthetic reasons are sometimes cited** for the operation, and this is occasionally said in other areas of Africa as well. It is claimed that a woman's external genitalia are ugly and must be removed to make her acceptable to a man.

Hypertrophy of the clitoris - which means an unusual enlargement of that organ which will, it is claimed, protrude between a woman's legs if not cut off - is cited as a reason for excision in Ethiopia and also in parts of Nigeria. The Catholic Church sanctioned the mutilation of all female children of its converts on those grounds, though **gynecologists working in Africa have never been able to find any evidence of this claim.**

Health reasons are often cited now, especially in urban areas where the traditional myths are forgotten. **Cleanliness is the reason given by middle class families** in areas as far apart as Cairo and Bamako. In Sudan, the operation is traditionally connected with cleanliness and is called "Tahur," which in Arabic means purity. **A woman is considered dirty and polluted unless she is mutilated.** The same is also often said in Somalia.

Many of the reasons given by local populations are quite similar, though they have been arrived at quite independently as no connection or communication exists between the population groups involved. Most myths about female sexuality in Africa and all over the world are shared by men, **which documents the amazing worldwide similarity of male attitudes concerning female sexuality**. Obviously, all of the myths are designed to justify and continue the operations, from which men derive power and control over women as a group. This is, of course, the real reason why these operations continue today and why they are being rapidly introduced into the modern sector throughout the African continent with the collusion of Western men, led by anthropologists who claim that Africans cannot be "deprived of their traditions." The male-dominated health system has forgotten the social rites and ceremonies: but the cutting continues because much money can be made by this surgery. The Health Minister of Egypt announced after the 1994 UN Population Conference in Cairo, where FGM was discussed, that he would set up a teaching program for physicians to do the operations in the hospitals.

Many different, fanciful stories are told about FGM in the ethnographic literature. One tale citing why clitoridectomy is practiced is related by Jacques Lantier as told to him by a witch doctor, **which has amazing contemporary relevance:**

> **"The great Spirit has created a woman in such a way** that he alone can create life in her at the moment of conception. The Spirit has never made anything without good reason. A woman has two different and separate areas where she experiences desire and excitement: the clitoris and the vagina. The vagina is closed and can't be opened until the husband, chosen by the ancestors, breaks the closure and thus makes a passage for the Spirit to enter and to continue the family. The Spirit decrees that this part of her body must not be soiled and he alone wants to give the woman the greatest possible pleasure. **The Spirit has given the woman a clitoris** so she can enjoy it before marriage and still remain pure. The pleasure she experiences will create in her a desire for marriage. One does not cut off the clitoris in small girls because they use it to masturbate. Only when they are ready to procreate is it removed; and once it is, they feel deprived. Their desire then is concentrated in one place only, and they promptly get married. The couple experiences great happiness as the Spirit said it should be." [14]

This story and similar ones are told by different African ethnic groups. But what is astonishing is that it **propagates the very same male myth of vaginal orgasm as the one prevalent among male medical professionals and followers of Freud.** Freud's misconceptions were accepted throughout the male-dominated educated Western world with the same reverence as the "wisdom" of the African witch doctor. Obviously, **neither Freud nor the African witch doctor were aware that they shared the same self-serving sexual myth of vaginal orgasm.** In both cases, women paid the price - in Africa, often with their lives. The most recent medical myth, propagated by an expatriate Sudanese physician, Nahid Toubia, **compared FGM to breast implants,** which she stated on a national television program in the US!

FGM is now performed on much younger children especially in urban areas, as girls may resist once they go to school or find out what really is done to them. Some run away - usually to the nearest towns. In 1991, one young woman from Mali went all the way to **Paris. Her family had thrown her out** when she refused to undergo excision prior to marriage as required traditionally in her village. She got permission to stay in France with the help of women lawyers. **But her mother paid the price, she was banned from her home and village as she was held responsible for her daughter's action.**

Today, the mutilations continue to be practiced even in families of government officials and political leaders even though many of the men have been to European or Western universities. The reason given by these men is "African tradition" - yet the men have rejected all other traditions for their own Westernized personal lives.

A few years ago, I interviewed a Somali delegate to a United Nations conference who replied that, yes, he had had all his daughters infibulated. "It is the custom - everyone does it," he said. This was after he had delivered a rousing speech on the efforts of the Somalian Government to modernize the country and to abolish traditions as they damaged his society!

It would be interesting to make a survey among African and Middle Eastern ambassadors and United Nations delegates - many of them polygamists - to learn the truth about their daughters. Many of these leaders, educated in Europe or the US, have adopted a Western lifestyle - clothes, cars, televisions, air-conditioned homes, jet travel, etc. Yet, as I learned, many subject their daughters to sexual mutilation despite the fact that the UN adopted the Children's Convention to globally protect children's lives and health. Why does the international diplomatic community not object to this criminal child abuse among their peers? **United Nations Secretary-General Boutros Boutros-Ghali is an Egyptian Copt: all Copts in Egypt practice excision. One can but wonder what is practiced in his family.**

In France, poor immigrant families are accused in criminal court of mutilating their children. All over the world FGM is prohibited as child abuse. Yet the African diplomats and leaders of their countries - **for instance, delegates at the United Nations in New York - may mutilate their own children, though it is a human rights violation according to the United Nations.** Not one African leader has ever publicly renounced the practice. No one has ever questioned the personal behavior of African and Middle Eastern leaders or how they treat their families.

GEOGRAPHIC DISTRIBUTION
EXCISION is practiced in a broad area all across Africa parallel to the Equator: from Egypt, Ethiopia, Somalia and Kenya in East Africa, to the West African coast, from Sierra Leone to Mauritania and in all countries in between, including Nigeria, the most populous one. Excision is also documented in the southern part of the Arab Peninsula and around the Persian Gulf, including Yemen, Oman, the Arab Emirates and Bahrain - where the operations are reported to be decreasing. The map shows the areas affected according to definite documentation. FGM is a traditional ethnic practice and has nothing to do with the political borders of Africa, which were drawn in the 19th century. A less damaging form of genital mutilation is traditionally practiced on Moslem girl-children in Malaysia and parts of Indonesia, where the practice was introduced with Moslemization; in Africa it is indigenous.

FGM is practiced today by some ethnic groups, most often by a majority of the inhabitants, **in more than 26 countries of the African continent.** However, there are exceptions. The Luo, the second largest ethnic group of Kenya and the political rivals of the dominant Kikuyu, do not operate on their girls or their boys - though they are surrounded by ethnic groups who do.

INFIBULATION is practiced on all females, almost without exception, in all of Somalia and wherever ethnic Somalis live (Ethiopia, Kenya and Djibouti). It is also performed throughout **Moslem Sudan and the Upper Nile Valley, including southern Egypt, Eritrea, parts of Ethiopia and all along the Red Sea coast.** The operation is traditionally performed on much younger children than is excision, usually on 4- to 8-year- old girls, long before puberty. Except for Sudan and Southern Egypt no ritual or celebration is involved.

In West Africa, infibulation is documented at the present time in **Mali** among some Moslem population groups. It is also practiced in **northern Nigeria** (Moslem area), according to a medical source, and is said to be practiced by some very traditional groups living along the river and in Eastern **Senegal.** No doubt infibulation is also practiced in other remote areas of West Africa. **Infibulation sometimes occurs spontaneously** as a result of extensive mutilations. This is reported in the medical literature from West Africa, including **Cote d'Ivoire** and **Burkina Faso,** where the operations are done in radical ways.

A worldwide survey on FGM was prepared by me for the World Health Organization seminar in 1979 on "Traditional Practices Affecting the Health of Women and Children" and published in the second volume of the seminar report. This survey is based on an extensive literature search and field work all over Africa. An updated version of this research was published a year later in my article, "Female Genital Mutilation in the World Today: A Global Review." [15]

EXCISION AND INFIBULATION IN AFRICA:

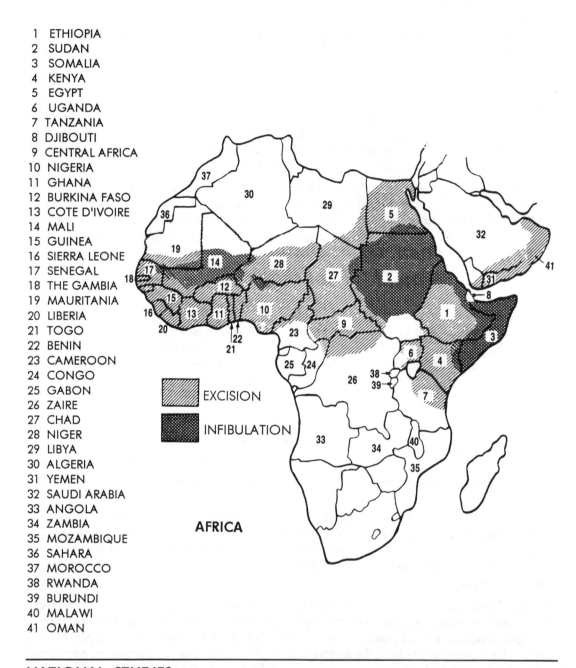

1   ETHIOPIA
2   SUDAN
3   SOMALIA
4   KENYA
5   EGYPT
6   UGANDA
7   TANZANIA
8   DJIBOUTI
9   CENTRAL AFRICA
10 NIGERIA
11 GHANA
12 BURKINA FASO
13 COTE D'IVOIRE
14 MALI
15 GUINEA
16 SIERRA LEONE
17 SENEGAL
18 THE GAMBIA
19 MAURITANIA
20 LIBERIA
21 TOGO
22 BENIN
23 CAMEROON
24 CONGO
25 GABON
26 ZAIRE
27 CHAD
28 NIGER
29 LIBYA
30 ALGERIA
31 YEMEN
32 SAUDI ARABIA
33 ANGOLA
34 ZAMBIA
35 MOZAMBIQUE
36 SAHARA
37 MOROCCO
38 RWANDA
39 BURUNDI
40 MALAWI
41 OMAN

EXCISION

INFIBULATION

AFRICA

NATIONAL STUDIES:

The most detailed national study was conducted in Sudan by Dr. Asma el Dareer of the medical faculty of the University of Khartoum. [16] In Nigeria, a national survey was made by the Federal Ministry of Health, Department of Medical Statistics, that showed that FGM is practiced in most Nigerian states. [17] . A study by Dr. Koso-Thomas in Sierra Leone established that the operations are practiced throughout the country. Partial surveys have been made in other countries, including Ghana, Kenya, Senegal, Egypt, Gambia, Liberia, and Chad. (See HOSKEN REPORT.) Due to population growth, urban immigration, civil wars and greater mobility, FGM is spreading to ever more and larger areas.

FEMALE GENITAL MUTILATION

ESTIMATE: TOTAL NUMBER OF GIRLS AND WOMEN MUTILATED IN AFRICA

Countries with Large % Mutilated	Total Population in Millions	Number of Women (50% of Total)	Percent Mutilated Women	Estimate Total in Millions
EAST AFRICA				
Egypt	61.64	30.82	60%	18.49
Sudan	27.36	13.68	85%	11.63
Somalia	9.08	4.54	99%	4.49
Djibouti	0.57	0.285	99%	0.28
Ethiopia	53.44	26.72	90%	24.05
Eritrea	3.44	1.72	80%	1.38
Kenya	27.34	13.67	60%	8.20

Total East Africa: 68.52 Mill

WEST AND CENTRAL AFRICA				
Nigeria	108.47	54.24	60%	32.54
Mali	10.46	5.23	75%	3.92
Burkina Faso	10.05	5.03	70%	3.52
Cote d'Ivoire	13.78	6.89	60%	4.13
Sierra Leone	4.4	2.2	90%	1.98
Guinea	6.5	3.25	70%	2.28
Guinea Bissau	1.05	0.525	70%	0.37
Togo	4.01	2.00	50%	1.00
Benin	5.25	2.63	50%	1.32
Chad	6.18	3.09	60%	1.85
Gambia	1.08	0.54	80%	0.43
Mauritania	2.22	1.11	40%	0.44
Ghana	16.94	8.47	30%	2.54
Liberia	2.94	1.47	70%	1.03
Senegal	8.10	4.05	20%	0.81
Central Africa	3.24	1.62	40%	0.65

TOTAL West and Central Africa: 58.81 Mill.

ESTIMATED NUMBER OF MUTILATED WOMEN AND GIRLS FOR CONTINENTAL AFRICA IN MILLIONS: 127.33 Mill.

In a number of other African countries, adjoining those cited above, a small percentage of the population practices FGM, which is **an ethnic custom regardless of political boundaries.** They include **Cameroon, Congo, Zaire, Tanzania, Uganda.** The total number of mutilated girls/ women is **estimated at 6-8 million.** This number should be added to the figures above, as well as the women/girls affected on the Arab peninsula. The estimated percentages are low and may be higher in some countries; they are computed based on the ethnic groups in each country known to practice FGM. (See appendix.) The population figures cited are from UNFPA statistics and need to be continuously updated as African populations grow 2.5-3% annually.   Copyright© 1995 Fran P. Hosken

FEMALE GENITAL MUTILATION OUTSIDE OF CONTINENTAL AFRICA

In the 14th century, Moslemization imported the operations into Malaysia and parts of Indonesia. In Asia, therefore, FGM is practiced only by devout Moslem families as a religious rite and never by any other ethnic or religious group. The operations in Asia are limited to a small cut of the prepuce or prick of the clitoris; they do not remove the organ or create hard scars. Childbearing is therefore not affected as in Africa though the cuts can cause infections and bleeding. Infibulation is never practiced in Asia.

At the 1988 UN conference in Mogadishu on "Strategies to Bring About Change," **a physician from Indonesia, a member of the medical faculty of Gadjah Mada University at Jogjakarta, presented his research on this subject**. His conclusion was that **at present the operations are carried out mostly as symbolic ceremonies,** and any surgical intervention "involves a light puncture of the tip of the clitoris." [18] But what is done in the many villages by traditional midwives who do the circumcision of girls has not been investigated. No adverse effects on childbirth are recorded, according to physicians.

In Malaysia, the operations are practiced by the Moslem Malays and not by any other ethnic group. In a recent study made in Malay villages the women stated that the practice consists in the removal of the prepuce of the clitoris; it is highly recommended by Islam for a female child. Recently, the ritual, which traditionally was a puberty rite to prevent promiscuity, is now being practiced on ever younger girls, sometimes immediately after birth. The village midwives did the operations in the past, but now to prevent infections the procedure is being medicalized and most of the former feasts and presents are omitted. The statements of the people asked in the study show that besides religious reasons it is believed that a girl's sexuality had to be controlled to make her a good Moslem woman. (See **The HOSKEN REPORT: Asia - Indonesia and Malaysia.**)

The idea that the genitalia of a girl must be cut, manipulated or altered to control her sexuality and make her acceptable to society, is an aberration, considering that **it is male sexuality that is violent and dangerous - it is men who rape**. But since men speak for society, **the danger that uncontrolled male sexuality represents has been transferred to women who are mutilated by male demand and made to pay for the sexual violence of men.**

A distinction must also be made between sporadic and isolated occurrences of the mutilations and the systematic subjection of all female children belonging to an ethnic group, as is the case in Africa. Recently, a researcher in Bombay, India, found that some members of **a Moslem sect in western India, the Bohras**, practice the sunna type of FGM - shrouded in strict secrecy. Apparently this group was converted to Islam by missionaries from Egypt who introduced this practice which is said to consist in nicking the clitoris, allegedly to curb female sexuality.[19] However, no medical corroboration exists.

In the medical literature, **several sporadic occurrences** of genital operations are cited outside of Africa or the Middle East. These citations are all from more than 100 years ago with no medical case histories to back them up; most are based on travelers' reports related as anecdotes in the anthropological literature. For instance, an operation called introcision (cuts into the vagina) is said to have been practiced in the 19th century among **the indigenous population of Australia**; no medical case histories exist, and reports from hospitals in the area confirm that the operations are quite unknown.

Another citation in the bibliographies of medical articles concerns a small group of **Orthodox monks in Czarist Russia called Skoptsi**, who are said to have practiced **self-castration of both men and women**. This undocumented story goes back to the first German edition of the anthropological study by Heinrich Ploss,[20] which was published in 1885. It was misinterpreted by some uninformed writers when the historic work of Ploss was translated into English in 1935, creating confusion ever since. It is possible that some isolated cases of genital operations as well as other damaging practices and taboos can be found among remote isolated communities, **but this has nothing to do with the systematic mutilation of all female children as absolute requirement on pain of expulsion from the family and group or what is practiced all over Africa and the Middle East today, involving more than 126 millions girls and women.**

The number of girls and women subjected to FGM outside of Africa is difficult to estimate. How many female children continue to be subjected to these operations in Malaysia or Indonesia cannot be established without field work - visiting Moslem hospitals, village dispensaries and maternity clinics. It would be necessary to travel all over the country and talk to local traditional midwives.

It is also difficult to estimate the number of women and girls mutilated in the southern part of the Arab Peninsula and along the Persian Gulf. It is unknown if the operations are practiced anywhere in Saudi Arabia or other Middle Eastern countries as mostly nomadic groups are involved who do not use hospitals and usually refuse all modern health care.

The mutilations, as stated before, now are also brought along by African and Middle Eastern immigrants, especially to **Europe and North America.** In this new environment all rituals and the pretext that this is an important tradition are gone, yet the surgery is continued on little girls even though it may ruin their lives and make them unacceptable to the people where they live. The reason is that immigrant men still require FGM for marriage. **Therefore all immigrants from Africa and especially men should be required to participate in education programs on reproductive health.**

EXCISION/INFIBULATION: EFFECT ON SEXUAL RESPONSE

In 1977, at the fifth Obstetrical-Gynaecological Congress in Khartoum, Sudan, Dr. Salah Abu Bakr showed a series of slides of the cell structure of specimens from the clitoris and labia minora of several girls, made from the parts cut off at an excision operation.[21] Seen through a microscope, the specimens, darkened by special dyes, revealed an abundance of nerve endings.

Dr. Bakr also showed similarly prepared slides made from the scar tissue of several adult women which was removed during repair operations; the few nerve endings that remained were encapsulated in sheets of fibrous tissue which renders them functionless. He explained, **"Excision and infibulation result in destruction of the nerve supply of the vulva; consequently, sexual arousal cannot take place."**

Touch organs (Pacinian corpuscles), Dr. Bakr stated, are removed by the operation, making the genital area insensitive to touch. Thus, it is physically impossible for a mutilated woman to be sexually stimulated by intercourse or respond to touch in the genital area.

Alternatively, some of the nerves may be accidentally bundled together by the cuts made during the operation and trapped in the scar tissue. As a result, touching such an area may become extremely painful, making sexual intercourse an excruciating ordeal.

This study by Dr. Bakr should lay to rest the claims made (often by male anthropologists) that the operations do not affect female sexual response. Without nerve endings, one cannot feel - much as without eyes, one cannot see. To ask women who have undergone FGM about their sexual experiences, as some researchers claim to have done, seems an exercise in futility. Worse, how can one explain orgasm to someone who has been mutilated as a child and associates the genital area with pain! As the groundbreaking study of **Dr. Shandall at the Khartoum Hospital established, sexual intercourse is frequently painful for women** who have undergone excision and infibulation, quite aside from the terrible ordeal of childbirth.[22] In view of these studies, claims made that excision and infibulation do not damage sexual response - allegedly based on interviews with Sudanese women - are obviously absurd. What is more, Sudanese women never talk about sexuality with strangers from abroad.

A FEMALE/MALE COMPARISON

The equivalent of excision/clitoridectomy is the excision of part or all of the penis. The equivalent of removing the tip of the clitoris (Sunna circumcision) is the same as the removal of the glans of the penis - both are most sensitive and full of nerve endings.

From the point of view of anatomy, **the clitoris and the penis are similar organs,** which is also confirmed by their embryonic development.

Fertility is not impaired by either excision of the clitoris or excision of the penis; production of semen by a man continues. Conception and pregnancy of a woman proceeds much the same in mutilated as in normal women. **Excision of the penis does not affect the production of sperm and semen,** anymore than excision of the clitoris affects ovulation. Children can be conceived by artificial insemination, which can be accomplished with simple tools, for instance, a spoon. The penis is not needed for fertilization.

Orgasm for men who have had penisectomies clearly is not possible, nor is it possible for women who have had clitoridectomies.

Penisectomy does not affect elimination of urine of the male, any more than clitoridectomy affects urination of the female, as soon as the wound is healed. But, while a man whose penis has been cut off experiences no other health problems after the wound has healed, the scars created by the female operation often result in terrible problems at childbirth. The tissues that must greatly stretch to let the baby come out are scarred and have lost their elasticity. **Obstructed labor, as a result of genital operations, costs many women and babies their lives after causing terrible suffering and agony due to tearing.**

It is claimed frequently in the literature written by men that Sunna circumcision (cutting off the tip of the clitoris) does no harm. **Sunna circumcision is the same operation as cutting off the tip or glans of the penis. Would men claim this does no harm ?** How would a man who claims that female circumcision does no harm like to have the most sensitive part of his body - the tip of his penis - cut off?

A discussion of male excision as an alternative to operating on females will make the issue quite clear. The option of introducing the female operation into modern health care was discussed at the 1979 WHO seminar in Khartoum by Sudanese physicians claiming this would "prevent worse harm." This option is also proposed repeatedly by Western male physicians, as is documented in **The HOSKEN REPORT,** and was again suggested in 1992 by physicians in the Netherlands who wanted to mutilate the infant daughters of Somalian refugees - at taxpayers' expense in government hospitals under the pretext to prevent "worse harm."

The former director of the population program of US Agency for International Development, Dr. R.T. Ravenholt, claimed that genital operations on females are "nothing but a traditional method of birth control." **It must be pointed out that male excision of the penis would be a much more effective method of birth control.**

Men in much of Africa and the Middle East claim that there is a "need" for excising females as a means of controlling their sexuality. **It is clear that the "need" for sexual control of males is much greater; rape and sexual assault are increasing all over the world, and male excision would certainly be a solution.** Furthermore, male excision would quite eliminate the "need" for female excision and would also greatly reduce the spread of AIDS.

Female sexual satisfaction is not dependent on penetration by the male penis: on the contrary, as was documented some time ago by Drs. Masters and Johnson [23] and in **The Hite Report.** [24] Female sexual satisfaction and orgasm are achieved by clitoral stimulation. Therefore, **female orgasm is quite independent of males and is not affected by excision of the penis. However, rape and sexual assault of women would be eliminated by penisectomies - which would be a very great benefit to all societies.**

Before the introduction of clitoridectomy into modern medical practice is further discussed, **male excision should be considered as a much more efficient alternative.** At the WHO seminar in Khartoum, the proposal to medicalize FGM by performing the operations in a hospital setting was voted down by all the women present; however, it has come up repeatedly since, always proposed by men, most recently in Cairo. Therefore, a comparative research study sponsored by WHO of the biological and health facts involved should be made to clarify the situation. **A cost benefit analysis of male excision (penisectomy) versus female clitoridectomy will, I predict, show the advantages of penisectomy, which will also eliminate rape.** No doubt such a study will raise the consciousness of men and should be presented to all politicians in Africa and the Middle East as well as to all physicians so keen to introduce FGM into hospital practice.

COST ANALYSIS

The terrible human costs of the operations cannot be measured, and are paid, first of all, by the young female children and women of Africa and the Middle East, sometimes with their lives.

The costs to governments, however, can be accounted for in monetary terms. By implication, these costs must also be faced by international agencies including those of the United Nations and all governments that finance development programs.*

There are four principal areas of costs involved:

1. **The costs due to loss of life of female children and young women** as the direct result of the operations. They represent an irretrievable loss to their own families, communities and each country.

2. **The costs of injuries, infections and of making childbirth more hazardous** as well as costs of lifelong health problems. With more women seeking help in the hospitals, the costs of health care are growing for each government. According to the regional office of WHO in Alexandria, it was estimated that during one year (July 1977-July 1978), in a single hospital of that region, 1,967 days of hospitalization were needed to care for those seeking help as a result of complications due to genital operations. "The costs are obviously high - especially in a developing country whose health resources are generally scarce." [25]

3. **The costs of work time lost due to illness,** including the recurring menstrual problems caused by the operations, that have to be borne by each employer. The largest employer in each African and Middle Eastern country is the government. When health insurance and social security arrangements are instituted, the costs of genital mutilations will have to be directly paid in health care costs by each insurer and by each government. These costs directly affect the development budget and the costs of development plans.

4. **The costs of introducing the operations into hospitals,** as some proposed, including the necessary drugs and care, would be well beyond the budget of any African or Middle Eastern country, especially since this means a continuously growing expense. By comparison, a national health education campaign to abolish these damaging practices would be a one-time expense. Such a budget is available for Sierra Leone, showing that it costs less to organize and run such a campaign over a 20-year period than the health costs involved in caring for the injured girls and women. Furthermore, the campaign would eliminate all future costs due to FGM. (See **The HOSKEN REPORT:** Sierra Leone.)

From this accounting, it is obvious that the costs faced now by organizing nationally and internationally supported health education and prevention campaigns to stop female genital mutilations will represent a very large net savings of direct expenses over the coming years. The emphasis should be on positive health and especially preventive health care. This is ever more urgent due to the growing disaster of AIDS to which FGM greatly contributes.

The objective is to eliminate genital mutilation and put in its place positive mother and child care practices through education in reproductive health, childbirth, child spacing, personal hygiene, nutrition, and more. Health education campaigns in family health directed to the whole family, especially women but also to male decision makers, will immeasurably improve the health and well-being of each country and community. Such campaigns will result in better health for the younger generation, and they will add up to a net reduction in health and medical budgets. **The Universal Childbirth Picture Book Program,** organized by Women's International Network, has proven to be a very effective teaching tool regardless of language or literacy.

---

* Development assistance is financed by taxes, which in turn are paid by all of us. **Therefore, we have a right to speak on how this money should be spent** and make our wishes known to the governmental agencies involved. In the United States, write to the Chief Administrator, USAID, Department of State, Washington, DC 20523.

FROM AN ADDRESS BY EDNA ADAN ISMAIL, WHO REPRESENTATIVE IN DJIBOUTI FORMER DIRECTOR OF TRAINING, HEALTH MINISTRY OF SOMALIA

"I thank you for having given me the opportunity to bring your attention to the subject of female genital mutilation. In various modifications, the operations rank high in the list of preventable health hazards . . . It may be appropriate here for me to describe more fully **the mental and physical injuries** and complications suffered by such a large number of our sisters and daughters.

After outlining the different types of operations, Ismail described the situation from her own experience working for many years as the director of midwifery and nurses training in the health ministry of Somalia. First, a description of the operation:

"The operations are carried out by women who earn their living by the performance of such operations, including the opening up, after marriage, of the bride; these women are also often the village midwives. Such women have no knowledge of asepsis or anatomy and use no form of anesthesia. **The operations may also be done by paramedical personnel**; such people use local anesthesia, sterile instruments and have some knowledge of the importance of asepsis. However, because of the local anesthesia, the child struggles less and more tissues may be cut away.

In Somalia, the operations are done on young girls between the ages of 5 and 8, and may be done on individuals or groups of girls, either related or neighbors. The child is made to squat on a stool or mat with a strong woman pinning back her arms and shoulders. Two more women each hold one of her legs and stop her from struggling.

The operator sits in front of the child, and with a razor blade or other sharp instrument excises the clitoris, labia minora and the inner walls of the labia majora. Using thorns which she has pre-selected, she inserts three or four on opposite sides of the labia majora, winds a string or a strip of cloth around the thorns in order to hold them together, very similar to how boots are laced. She then sprinkles the wound with a powder mixed from sugar, gum and myrrh. This forms a glue and sticks to the cloth, thorns and blood and forms a crust which stops the bleeding. **The child is then bound from the waist to her toes and is made to lie on her side on a mat.**

Aftercare depends on the type of operations performed. In Somalia, it may consist of the cauterization of the wound, the application of herbs which are believed to have haemostatic properties and enhance healing. The girls' diet is restricted in order to prevent frequent bowel movements, and her drinking is also limited to a few sips of water at a time. Fumigations are frequent in order to dispel any undesirable odors and evil spirits."

Next, Ismail reviews the many health problems including the resulting mental trauma based on her own experience as a trained midwife and teacher of midwifery:

"As you can imagine, **there are many complications; shock from fear, pain and hemorrhage.** Extensive lacerations may be sustained which may involve the vaginal and urethral openings, as well as sometimes the rectum. The hemorrhages may be so severe that quite a few children are brought into the hospital for suturing of deep lacerations and for blood transfusions.

Within the first 10 days, sepsis ranks high in the list of complications and tetanus may also result. Retention of urine is another common complication due to the fact that the urethra is now covered with a flap of skin, thorns and blood clots, as well as the swelling which develops and obstructs the small opening which has been left to permit the passage of urine. Failure of the infibulation means that the walls of the labia majora fail to stick together. Another attempt at infibulation is usually made.

At the time of marriage, the forcible penetration of the skin barrier by the husband may cause lacerations, which may involve the perineum, the urethra, and sometimes even the rectum - particularly if a knife is used by the husband. **At childbirth, the scars of the external genitalia have very little elasticity** and require being opened up in order to permit the passage of the baby through the obstructed birth outlet. Once more, infections may occur. This unnecessary suffering is imposed on the woman during every childbirth.

At the time of marriage, the forcible penetration of the skin barrier by the husband may cause lacerations, which may involve the perineum, the urethra, and sometimes even the rectum - particularly if a knife is used by the husband.

At childbirth, the scars of the external genitalia have very little elasticity and require being opened up in order to permit the passage of the baby through the obstructed birth outlet. Once more, infections may occur. This unnecessary suffering is imposed on the woman during every childbirth.

Other complications are rectovaginal and vesico-vaginal fistulae - the rupture of the vagina resulting in incontinence. Cystocoles, which is the prolapse of the bladder, the rectum and the uterus, are common. Pelvic inflammation also occurs due to the retention of urine and menstrual blood in the vagina and urethra. There is a constant threat of cystitis, vaginitis, cervicitis, and other infections which may develop into a chronic pelvic inflammation leading to dysmenorrhea (painful menstruation) and infertility.

Mental complications begin to affect the female child from an early age, and remain with her throughout her life. Well before the child is operated on, she hears tales of horror relating to the act of infibulation. **At the same time, girls who have undergone FGM taunt those who have not with insults and call them 'unclean.'** In this frame of mind, of fear mixed with a sense of inferiority, the girl reaches her turn for the surgery. Many of the physical wounds will heal; their pain and discomfort subside. But at each stage of her later life further mental injuries are added.

The slow trickle of urine (as opposed to the strong jet of urine coming from her bladder) reminds her constantly of the operation. The onset of menstruation, with its accompanying discomfort and odors, forces her to recall her agony. Marriage and the opening up of the infibulation to permit the consummation of the marriage is an ordeal. **The birth of the first child and the knowledge that subsequent deliveries are not going to be any easier on her scar-riddled genitals, constantly haunt every woman.**
In spite of her own suffering due to infibulation, the knowledge that she will have to subject her daughters to the same ordeal adds further to her mental agonies." [26]

Edna Adan Ismail was the first woman and health professional to speak in public in Somalia on the health problems resulting from excision and infibulation when she addressed the congress of the **Somali Democratic Women's Organization (SWDO)** in March 1977. The 500 participants attending the Congress unanimously condemned the practice and **expressed their support for abolishment.** This led to the formation of a National Commission to Abolish Female Circumcision under the guidance of the SWDO and gained the support of the president of Somalia and the ministries of health, education, and religious guidance.

In Somalia, FGM has always been practiced in the extreme form of infibulation, according to the earliest reports available, and this continues today involving almost the entire female population - with terrible results - as Ismail describes above. It is, therefore, quite remarkable that in a few years after the 1979 Khartoum seminar, where a large delegation from Somalia participated including Ismail, **the most comprehensive program to eradicate FGM was organized.** It began to be implemented in 1986-87 by the government led by the SWDO with the collaboration and financial as well as technical support by the Italian Association for Women in Development (AIDoS). [27]

This effort had the full backing of President Mohamed Siad Barree, who had been in power since 1969. All ministries and the entire school system participated in this groundbreaking national program. Besides organizing local and national meetings to mobilize leaders on every level as well as running education and training programs of all kinds, **it culminated in an international conference in June 1988, organized by the SWDO and AIDoS jointly and held in the Parliament.** [28]

This unique international meeting - nothing like it had ever been done before or since anywhere in Africa - was publicized and broadcast all over Somalia, where until recently FGM was never discussed. At the time of the conference in Mogadishu, the political upheaval that now engulfs the whole country had already started in the north.

A growing famine added to the ever wider civil war which began to threaten the very existence of the majority of the people. International assistance involving the US and United Nations troops became the target of the local warlords, who hijacked and used food shipments to gain power **exposing their own women and children to starvation.** Somali men continue their clan warfare today, after destroying their own country. Women and children are the victims of these endless power struggles which will no doubt continue until the last bullet is spent. Violence is all these men know, which starts in the family by brutalizing their own small daughters through infibulation and indoctrinating their sons into a life where destruction of all others is the only measure of success of each clan.

The Somalian initiative and program to eradicate infibulation, entirely organized by women, however, can serve as a model and an inspiration. The educational materials, including videotapes and programs developed by AIDoS, are now being adapted and used in Ethiopia, Gambia, Nigeria and Sudan by their national committees affiliated with the IAC. (See **The HOSKEN REPORT**: Women and Health.)

FOOTNOTES

1. Women's International Network-**WIN NEWS**, "an open participatory quarterly journal by, for and about women," began publication in 1975 and reports on women's development from all regions of the world. Editor/publisher Fran P. Hosken, 187 Grant St., Lexington, MA 02173. **WIN NEWS** has had a section on FGM since 1975.

2. Hosken, Fran P. **The Childbirth Picture Book/Program,** "A picture story of reproduction from a woman's view"; pictures by Marcia L. Williams. Published since 1980 by Women's International Network News (address above). Books, flipcharts, color slides in English, French, Spanish, Arabic (also printed in India in six languages, in Nepal and the Marshall Islands). Additions to Prevent Excision and Infibulation in English, French and Arabic. Nutrition supplements in English, French and Spanish. For community health workers and families worldwide.

3. **The Inter-African Committee on Traditional Practices Affecting the Health of Women and Children.** c/o Economic Commission for Africa, ATRCW, P.O. Box 3001, Addis Ababa, Ethiopia. Inter-African Committee, 147, rue de Lausanne, CH-1202 Geneva, Switzerland.

4. Widstrand, Carl Gosta. "Female Infibulation," **Studia Ethnographica Upsaliensa,** Vol. XX, 1964.

5. Thiam, Awa. **La Parole Aux Negresses.** Denoel/Gonthier, 19 rue de l'Universite, 75007 Paris, France, 1978.

6. "College of Physicians and Surgeons of Ontario, Canada, Prohibits Female Genital Mutilation." 80 College St., Toronto M5G 2E2, Canada. See **WIN NEWS** Vol. 18, No. 2, Spring 1992, p. 46.

7. "Female Genital Mutilation - Is It Practiced in the USA?" See **WIN NEWS** Vol.16, No. 33, Summer 1990, pp. 28-30; from **American Medical News,** April 27,1990, published by the American Medical Association.

8. United Nations Center for Human Rights, CH-1211 Geneva, Switzerland. "UN Seminar on Traditional Practices Affecting the Health of Women and Children." E/CN.4/SUB.2/1991/48 12. June 1991. April 29-May 3,1991, Ouagadougou, Burkina Faso. See **WIN NEWS** Vol.17, No. 3, p. 31 and 17-4 pp. 29-31.

9. Shandall, Ahmed Abu-El Futuh, M.D. "Circumcision and Infibulation of Females," **Sudan Medical Journal,** Vol. 5, No. 4, December 1967.

10. Cook, Robert, M.D. Regional MCH-Nut Advisor, World Health Organization, Regional Office for the Eastern Mediterranean, P.O. Box 1517, Alexandria, Egypt. "Damage to Physical Health from Pharaonic Circumcision (Infibulation) of Females: A Review of the Medical Literature," 1976.

11. Verzin, J.A., M.D. "Sequelae of Female Circumcision," **Tropical Doctor,** October 1975.

12. Baasher, T.A., Dr. (Frc Psych). "Psychological Aspects of Female Circumcision." Regional Advisor on Mental Health, World Health Organization, EMRO, P.O. Box 1517, Alexandria, Egypt.

13. Kenyatta, Jomo. **Facing Mount Kenya**. Vintage Books, Division of Random House, New York, October 1965.

14. Lantier, Jacques. **La Cite Magique et Magie en Afrique Noire**. Librarie Fayard, 1972.

15. Hosken, Fran P. "Female Circumcision in the World Today: A Global Review," **Traditional Practices Affecting the Health of Women and Children**, WHO/EMRO Technical Publication No. 2, Vol. 2, 1982 (Background Papers to the WHO Seminar), pp.195-214. The same article was revised and published as "Female Genital Mutilation in the World Today: A Global Review," published in **International Journal of Health Services**, Vincente Navarro, Editor-in-Chief, Baywood Publishing Co., 120 Marine St., P.O. Box D, Farmingdale, NY 11735 (Vol. 11, No. 3, 1981, pp. 415-30).

16. El Dareer, Asma Abdel Rahim, M.D., Dept. of Community Medicine, Faculty of Medicine, University of Khartoum, Sudan. **"An Epidemiological Study of Female Circumcision in the Sudan,"** thesis submitted for the degree of M.Sc. in Community Medicine, 1980/81. See also **WIN NEWS**, Vol. 7, No. 2, Spring 1981, p. 37 and Vol. 7, No. 3, Summer 1981, pp. 38-39.

17. "Final Report on Position of Female Circumcision in Nigeria," signed by Dr. O.A. Adelaja, Sr., consultant, Medical Statistics, Federal Ministry of Health, Fed. Secretariat, Ikoyi, Lagos, Nigeria (March 1981). See **WIN NEWS,** Vol. 7, No. 3, p. 41.

18. Pratiknya, Ahmad Watik. Prof., Faculty of Medicine, Gadjah Mada University, Yogyakarta, Indonesia. "Female Circumcision in Indonesia: A Synthesis Profile of Cultural, Religious and Health Values," pp. 51-56. **Female Circumcision: Strategies To Bring About Change**. Proceedings of the Seminar on Female Circumcision, 13-16 June 1988, Mogadishu, Somalia. Published by AIDoS - Italian Association or Women in Development, Via dei Giubbonari, 30 - 00186 Rome, Italy.

19. Ghadially, Rehana, Dept. of Humanities, Indian Institute of Technology, Bombay, 76 India. "The Practice of Female Circumcision Among the Bohra Muslims of India," **WIN NEWS** Vol. 18, No. 2, Spring 1992, p. 45.

20. Ploss, Heinrich, **Das Weib**. 1885 (first edition in German). Also, Ploss and Bartels, **Das Weib** 1886-1908 (second through ninth editions in German).

21. Bakr, Salah Abu, M.D. "Circumcision and Infibulation in the Sudan: Its Effect on the Innervation of the Vulva," paper presented at the fifth Obstetrical/Gynaecological Congress, Khartoum, Sudan, 1977. (Copy in author's file.)

22. Shandall, op. cit.

23. Masters & Johnson, **Human Sexual Response**, Little Brown Co., 1966.

24. Hite, Shere. **The Hite Report**, Dell Publishing Co., Inc., New York, 1976.

25. Taba, A.H., M.D. "Female Circumcision," **World Health,** World Health Organization, 1211 Geneva 27, Switzerland, May 1979, p. 10.

26. Report of the World Conference of the U.N. Decade for Women: Equality, Development and Peace, Copenhagen, July 14-30, 1980. Document #A/CONF. 94/35, p. 34.

27. AIDoS - Italian Association for Women and Development. Via dei Giubbonari 30 - 00186 Rome, Italy. Daniela Colombo, director.

28. **"Female Circumcision: Strategies to Bring About Change"** - Proceedings of International Seminar on Female Circumcision, June 13-16, 1988. Mogadishu, Somalia. Report by AIDoS. (See above.) See **WIN NEWS** Vol. 14, No. 3, pp. 28-31.

THE POLITICS OF FEMALE GENITAL MUTILATION

THE CONTEXT: DISCRIMINATION AT THE UNITED NATIONS

"Women are fifty percent of the world's adult population and one third of the official labor force; they perform two thirds of the actual working hours for which they receive one-tenth of the world's income and they own less than one percent of the world's property."*

The Convention on the Elimination of Discrimination Against Women (CEDAW),** which has been ratified by most African countries where Female Genital Mutilation (FGM) is practiced, protects each woman's integrity and right to control her own body. FGM is internationally recognized as a human rights violation. (See chapter on "Human Rights.") All countries that have signed on to CEDAW are required to regularly file progress reports on their efforts to implement the rights spelled out in the Convention. These accounts provide a vivid picture of the discrimination and injustices to which women are subjected under the jurisdiction of male-dominated governments.

Where the breach of the clauses of the Convention is too blatant and the prevailing practices too obviously against the agreements signed by the governments, the decision makers - all men - simply declare this area of the law to be exempt, or outside all scrutiny. The United Nations, which is supposed to support the implementation of all international agreements, is a body of governments run by men intent on protecting their own male privileges, and so they do nothing. Only about 3.4 percent of decision-making positions at the UN and its agencies are held by women, according to the reports of the Statistical Office of the UN Secretariat in New York.

The UN and its agencies do not recognize equal employment rules for women, though all the governments that financially support the UN system have long since implemented such legislation, because their women voters have demanded it. But the male-dominated governments have taken care to omit equal employment rules for the UN **while loudly proclaiming the benefits of democratic institutions which they deny to women** - half the population of the world. Consequently, the UN and all its agencies including all those working in Africa are bastions of male privilege and discrimination. Women working in the UN and international agencies have no protection against sexual assault, as documented by the Claxton case at the UN Secretariat in New York. (See **WIN NEWS**, Vol. 21, No. 2, Spring 1995, p. 9.)

Many of the men who work for UN agencies as well as diplomats are from Africa. They have their own daughters mutilated and never speak for women's rights as this would undermine their own power and privileges at home, where "their" women are still under absolute male control. Many are also polygamists. **Since most international civil servants are men they keep silent** in solidarity with their African and Middle Eastern colleagues and thus are protecting discrimination and FGM.

The US and all governments that make financial contributions to the UN and its agencies have had equal employment laws in place for decades. Why, then, don't they require that these agencies provide equal job opportunities for women, since these contributions come from taxes including those paid by women? **At present, women are all but excluded from decision-making jobs with devastating results for development.** The absence of women especially in UN offices in developing countries has resulted in blatant discrimination in program development for women, which is especially critical where health is concerned. The failure of the World Health Organization (WHO) and UNICEF to effectively deal with FGM is documented in detail in the chapter on "Politics" in **The HOSKEN REPORT** and is summarized below.

---

*Statement summarizing the status of Women from the UN Mid-Decade Conference.
**Convention on the Elimination of Discrimination Against Women, United Nations Division for the Advancement of Women, 2 UN Plaza, DC2-1220, N.Y., NY 10017.

THE CONSPIRACY OF SILENCE

The conspiracy of silence was first officially broken in 1979 by the WHO seminar in Khartoum, followed by the organization in 1984 of the **Inter-African Committee on Traditional Practices Affecting the Health of Women and Children (IAC)**. By now FGM is freely discussed in most of Africa, which is a major breakthrough. However, the resistance to deal with the issue by many working internationally, especially in health and population, continues. As with all issues that affect women, initiating action is met by resistance and unwillingness to change. Nevertheless, it is no longer possible to claim, as was done especially by UN agencies including WHO and UNICEF as well as by most NGOs working in Africa and church groups, that "FGM is practiced in a few remote areas by some isolated groups." Or, as the UNICEF information director in New York had told me after returning from an extended research trip to sub-Saharan Africa in 1973, **UNICEF had no information about such practices and "could not interfere in cultural traditions."**

What is astonishing is that none of the health professionals working for WHO and UNICEF or for the many charitable organizations and church groups that also maintain hospitals in Africa, ever published any information on FGM. It is difficult to understand the motivations of **health care professionals who, as the record shows, deliberately ignored major health problems that damage the lives and health of millions of girls and women** and their families as well as the economies of many African countries. This, quite aside from the terrible suffering and pain inflicted on innocent victims who are denied both the information and care they need.

Why did these men - and **international health is still an almost entirely male-dominated activity** - keep these problems silent? How is it possible for a responsible person, let alone a health professional who knows the consequences of his silence, to act in this way? WHO, UNICEF, the many church groups and USAID have enormous resources available and have access to communication which enables them to introduce and support change. Instead, they kept the problem hidden, evading their responsibilities. And even now, they are reluctant to make available the necessary resources.

When I first began to learn about **the unwillingness of the international health officials to speak the truth about FGM,** I tried to publish the facts. At that time, 20 years ago, most people in the Western world, and especially women, knew nothing about the issue and many were quite unwilling to believe the truth. I found that newspapers and magazines were quite unwilling to publish any articles on the subject and simply rejected all reports, though my work on other topics was regularly accepted and printed.

Even now, there is a continuing unwillingness to accept the facts on the part of many organizations working in Africa today in health and population; most of the major programs are funded by USAID (see below). Though FGM is now openly discussed in most African countries and some major efforts are underway to prevent and eradicate FGM, the unwillingness to either face the facts or to support the efforts by African groups and organizations such as the **IAC** continues.

What is the reason, at this stage, when the dimensions of the problem of FGM are known to anyone working in health in Africa, to continue to pretend that FGM is no problem, which is still the case among international health professionals? How can one ignore this terrible, preventable torture and suffering that the international health community is able to change? Are these international health officials afraid of African men, or what is the reason for this continuing the denial?

The interest of African men who have their daughters mutilated is quite clear - it is control over women, a higher brideprice and the approval by other men in their communities.

The interest of those who earn a living from doing the mutilations in traditional communities is also clear as well as the motivations of those in the health sector in Africa - both men and women - who do the operations in clinics and hospitals for money. Indeed there are some people so misguided as to claim that it is better to do the operations the medical way, **though this is obviously a violation of medical ethics.**

But how can the many population organizations and international family planning programs that work in Africa claim that they introduce contraception to save women's lives and then refuse to acknowledge that FGM damages both women's lives and health, denying women and families the education about FGM they so urgently need?

But the denial of FGM is continued by all the initiatives to promote "Safe Motherhood." There are millions spent on high-level meetings, conferences and research conducted by physicians sitting in their offices at WHO in Geneva or at US universities, but FGM is never mentioned. Obstructed labor was identified from the beginning as one of the six major causes of death in childbirth; and it is cited especially in Africa. But the fact that obstructed labor is most of all caused by FGM has not been mentioned at all though the highest per capita death rates in childbirth are recorded in sub-Saharan Africa, in the regions where FGM is practiced.

Silence is also maintained by all organizations and programs on "Safe Motherhood" active in Africa today. It must be greatly applauded that this terrible annual death toll of women in childbirth - most of them in developing countries - has finally attracted world attention and concern. But it is outrageous that the organizations and agencies dealing with the problem continue to suppress information that FGM is one of the major causes of childbirth mortality in sub-Saharan Africa.

All this is documented and detailed in **The HOSKEN REPORT** in the chapter on "Politics."

But the silence about FGM continues in the highest diplomatic circles, including and especially at the UN.

The current Secretary-General of the UN, Boutros Boutros-Ghali, is from the Coptic community of Egypt, where FGM is the rule, as documented in **The HOSKEN REPORT** (see "Case History: Egypt"). Since FGM was discussed at the UN population conference in Cairo in 1994, Boutros-Ghali should be questioned by the press as to how many girls of his own extended family are mutilated. The Egyptian Government, after CNN showed an excision operation videotaped in a home in Cairo during the conference, stated that FGM would be prohibited. But after the conference closed they reversed their position. FGM is being medicalized, that is, introduced into hospitals. **This means the mutilation of girls will be paid for by the Egyptian Government, and this government receives huge contributions from US taxpayers as voted by Congress.**

THE US AND US AGENCY FOR INTERNATIONAL DEVELOPMENT (USAID)

According to the American Overseas Interest Act, Egypt is to receive $2.1 billion in aid in the next fiscal year. **Congresswomen Patricia Schroeder*** inserted the following Resolution on FGM in this legislation which was passed June 7, 1995:

> "Whereas, female genital mutilation is a violation of women's basic human rights; and
>
> Whereas, female genital mutilation constitutes a major health risk to women, with lifelong physical and psychological consequences; and
>
> Whereas, female genital mutilation should not be condoned by any government;
>
> **It is the sense of Congress that:**
>
> The President seeks to end the practice of female genital mutilation worldwide through the active cooperation and participation of governments in whose nations female genital mutilation takes place. Steps to end the practice of female genital mutilation shall include:
>
> (1) encouraging nations to establish clear policies against female genital mutilation, and enforcing existing laws which prohibit it; and
>
> (2) assisting nations in creating culturally appropriate outreach programs that include education and counseling about the dangers of female genital mutilation for women and men of all ages; and
>
> **(3) ensuring that all appropriate programs in which the U.S. participates include a component pertaining to female genital mutilation, so as to ensure consistency across the spectrum of health and child related programs conducted in any country in which female genital mutilation is known to be a problem."**

---

*Congresswoman Patricia Schroeder, 2208 Rayburn Bldg., Washington, DC 20515

In the press release accompanying the resolution these statements are made:

"Schroeder's resolution was prompted in part by the Egyptian Government's move to medicalize FGM. On Oct. 29, **Egyptian Health Minister Ali Abdel Fatah issued a decree designating certain hospitals to perform the operation for about $3 U.S.** The decree represented a turnaround by the minister, who publicly stated at the United Nations International Conference on Population and Development in Cairo last September that FGM should be banned and those who performed it punished . . .

"Schroeder's sense of Congress resolution was part of an en bloc amendment offered by Rep. Benjamin Gilman, R-N.Y., to the American Overseas Interests Act, which authorizes foreign aid. The amendment passed on a voice vote. **The act earmarked $ 2.1 billion in aid for Egypt** . . .

"Schroeder is the sponsor of H.R. 941, the Federal Prohibition of Female Genital Mutilation Act of 1995, which criminalizes FGM for girls younger than 18 and requires Health and Human Services to identify and educate communities in this country that practice FGM, make recommendations to medical schools for treatment of its complications and compile statistics on women living here who have undergone it. Schroeder introduced a similar bill last Congress."

The question must be raised with USAID, which has financed extensive health and population programs all over Egypt: since $3 obviously does not cover the cost of the operations, **how is the Agency going to make sure that the US contributions are not going to be used to subsidize the mutilation of Egyptian girls in the hospitals?**

The resolution by Schroeder addresses the very same critical points that I have made since 1980 in my congressional testimonies before the Foreign Operations Subcommittee of the Appropriations Committee, which deals with funding of USAID and foreign assistance on the Senate side (for a copy, write to **WIN NEWS**). I urged that FGM prevention should be integrated especially in all ongoing US-funded population and health programs in Africa where FGM is practiced, which could be done immediately at little or no extra cost. I also proposed that the Inter-African Committee* and its affiliates in each country should be invited to join the AID-funded programs as consultants.

My testimony states:

> **"We urge that USAID and their contractors be required to integrate FGM prevention in all their population, family planning and health plans and programs** in FGM-affected countries and that every support be provided to local groups in Africa working for FGM prevention, for instance, the affiliates of the IAC are now active in 25 African countries . . .

> There is no reason why US-funded programs in Africa should not discourage FGM and teach about the unnecessary damage done to girls and women - especially since by now **FGM is discussed everywhere in Africa.** All USAID contractors and private organizations receiving USAID funds should be required to provide reports on their actions to prevent FGM and document results of the effectiveness of their teaching.

> **Similarly, all organizations receiving funding and contributions by the US including UNICEF, WHO, UNFPA (United Nations Population Fund), IPPF (International Planned Parenthood Federation)** and other organizations working in international health and development should be held responsible for integrating preventive education and accountable for results. To continue to ignore FGM results in the medicalization of these damaging practices in the modern sector - as has already happened in many towns in Africa. . ."

The Foreign Operations Subcommittee also votes on contributions for the United Nations and its agencies including UNICEF, WHO, UNFPA and all other international governmental programs.

---

*Inter-African Committee (IAC), 147, rue de Lausanne, CH-1202 Geneva, Switzerland.

USAID has a long history of failed programs in Africa, especially concerning health and population, in many sub-Saharan countries where FGM is practiced. The Agency and its many nongovernmental contractors in the health and population field (contracts are awarded based on competitive bids and experience) have over the years deliberately ignored FGM even if it is practiced in the very areas where family planning programs are implemented. The fact that girls and women are mutilated, for instance, all over Kenya has been all along deliberately ignored. Yet US-funded family planning clinics that examine women, of course, all know the facts.

It is astonishing that even now where FGM is widely discussed in Africa by Africans, USAID and their contractors have remained silent about the terrible health damage done to girls and women. They are doing nothing at all to prevent it or to teach the facts about reproductive health as, for instance, the **Childbirth Picture Books** do, which are published and distributed by **WIN NEWS.** They graphically show the physical damage done by the mutilations in a way that can be understood regardless of literacy (see Appendix).

Many international organizations continue to hide behind "culture," claiming they cannot interfere in tradition though **the IAC and their many affiliated groups as well as local people in many African countries are trying to stop FGM** where it is practiced, and are organizing prevention programs, which are ignored by USAID and their contractors. This disregard of women's health puts in doubt the very motivation by population programs which evidently are just another way for male-dominated international organizations to control women's bodies with no regard for women's needs.

The implemention of population programs contributes directly to the medicalization of FGM. These programs train local people in medical procedures, but they fail to teach against FGM. **Therefore these newly acquired skills by local people are often used to perform the mutilations the medical way for money,** which is not discouraged by the international contractors who run the programs, claiming they cannot interfere.

In most towns and all capitals in Africa the mutilations are now being medicalized, while the very people who provide the training and resources keep silent, thus supporting the medicalization and modernization of FGM. And this goes on with the full knowledge of USAID as provider of funds, training and antibiotics and with the collaboration of all their contractors in Africa. This I have not only protested at AID for years, but pointed out repeatedly in my congressional testimonies, which have been completely ignored (see **The HOSKEN REPORT,** "Women and Health," pp. 412-413).

As documented in Egypt (see above) and as the experience in Sudan over many years confirms, **physicians in Africa and the Middle East are only too willing to engage in this lucrative trade and take advantage of the opportunity to mutilate children to make money.** And this goes on with the full knowledge of the men who run USAID.*

But what is even more disturbing is that those who manage this agency (Congress voted AID a budget of over $580 million just for population programs for the 1995 fiscal year) **are now spreading false rumors in Washington that USAID has and is funding the IAC including their conferences.**

For instance, Richard McCall, chief of staff, was cited in an article that appeared in 1994 in the **Washington Post,** stating that "the Agency helped pay for a conference on FGM that was held in Ethiopia."** However, the facts are that even now, a year after this was published, **AID has not provided a cent for this conference, held in Addis Ababa by the IAC in spring of 1994,** so states Berhane Ras-Work, IAC president, despite repeated promises personally made by McCall. The "creative funding mechanism" that McCall claims AID has applied regarding funding of FGM prevention - as cited in the article by Judy Mann, who evidently fell for the hoax - turns out to be nothing but misleading posturing. Nor has USAID ever provided any effective support to any FGM prevention program in Africa.

---

*Contact J. Brian Atwood, Administrator, USAID, 320 21st St., N.W., Washington, DC 20523 and Richard McCall, Chief of Staff.

Washington Post, April 29, 1994, "From Victims to Agents of Change," by Judy Mann, p. E3.

Misleading the public by publishing articles in the Washington Post and making false promises to African women, as McCall did to the president of the IAC, **is adding insult to the torture and the human rights violations USAID and its staff have so long ignored.** On top of that, a representative of the Global Bureau of USAID, Ambassador Sally Shelton, announced at the National Conference for International Health in June 1995, in Washington, that AID is funding the IAC, which is completely untrue. According to Ras-Work, who was a speaker at the same conference at a panel discussion on FGM which I arranged and moderated, the IAC has never received any contribution from AID or their contractors.

It is astonishing that **although I pointed out to both McCall and Shelton that what they claimed publicly has been proven to be false, this fact has been entirely ignored,** and AID - our public servants - are evidently able to get away with it. One can but wonder how many other lies are told and promises broken by these bureaucrats, who evidently believe that since this affects women they can do and claim most anything. Congress recently has threatened to shut down AID; it certainly is high time to set new priorities.

As this book goes to press, just before the Fourth United Nations World Conference on Women in Beijing, women in the US should understand that **USAID, their government's agency concerned with international development and required by law to observe equal opportunity, has let them down and worse. AID has desperately damaged women all over the developing world** by their unwillingness to listen to women or women's real concerns and needs.

The record of USAID - as I have seen for myself in Africa - is appalling, especially where women and health programs are concerned, as I have documented in my congressional testimonies over the years, which are all available and on record. I cannot keep silent about the damage done to women and girls. Women and their children have been ignored, excluded, lied to and insulted by USAID and its personnel, as the examples cited above show, and this must change.

The US has always had the largest budget for foreign aid and development of any country, especially for population and health. Therefore, the Agency must be held responsible for the needless deaths and torture of millions of girls and women due to keeping FGM secret for years and its failure to support effective prevention and eradication of FGM. Women taxpayers in the US should demand a public accounting and hold personally responsible the men who run this mismanaged self-serving enterprise.

THE REACTIONS AND INITIATIVES OF WHO AND UNICEF

WHO and UNICEF are the two largest international institutions concerned with health, and, in the case of UNICEF specifically, with children's health. WHO is an international organization of health ministries. **The health ministers of virtually all governmental health departments all over the world are members.** Health ministry delegations meet every year in early spring in Geneva, at the WHO headquarters, where global health policies are developed.

UNICEF, by comparison, is an organization that works on the local level, assisting and helping to organize local programs for children or mothers with small children, including immunizations and initiatives against childhood diseases, all kinds of child care education, nutrition programs, and much more. **UNICEF gets large annual contributions from governments but raises money from the private sector as well** - for instance, by organizing various fundraising programs such as its greeting cards. There are UNICEF support groups in all Western countries that raise funds. Both WHO and UNICEF have offices in every country with local staff, headed by international administrators who usually rotate every few years to different countries and assignments.

WHO also has regional offices in different parts of the world. Africa is divided between the Regional Office of the Mediterranean, located in Alexandria, Egypt, and the WHO AFRO office in Brazzaville, Congo.

Both agencies work on local programs with local people in the countries they serve and enjoy international diplomatic privileges. **Most of the decision makers are men. There are almost no women in charge of country offices of WHO; the vast majority of UNICEF administrators overseas are also men** even though UNICEF's mandate is to serve children. The pervasive discrimination against women practiced even today by the international institution throughout the UN system, has devastating results for the women in developing countries, as I have seen for myself repeatedly by visiting their offices all over Africa.

How else is it possible that these two large, influential and prestigious organizations that are recognized and supported all over the world, have so utterly failed to address FGM, which damages the lives and health of more than 127 million girls and women in a huge region of the world? By any definition, **FGM must be classified as a major regional public health problem, affecting many tens of millions of families.**

Both of these powerful international agencies, charged with health around the world, have refused for many years to acknowledge even the existence of FGM or deal with the health problems resulting from these damaging mutilations. What is more, how could these agencies, supported by public funds and voluntary contributions in order to serve people around the world - especially children for UNICEF - **intentionally conceal for such a long time the ongoing mutilation of millions of little girls,** including the terrible permanent health damage of women that results?

But now, the secrecy has been broken and the information about FGM cannot be hidden any longer because African women have taken up the issue and are organizing in most African and Middle Eastern countries where FGM is practiced. Women are working all over Africa to stop this violent interference in the normal reproductive process. Both agencies certainly are experienced in organizing all kinds of health information campaigns with positive results - the small pox eradication campaign by WHO and the child-immunization campaigns of UNICEF are excellent and successful examples. **Why have these agencies failed to take some of the most urgent and necessary actions to initiate information and education campaigns against FGM or support those that exist?**

Both UNICEF and WHO have jointly organized the recent **grass roots campaigns on oral rehydration,** which was and is very successful and has saved countless children's lives. Over the years, **WIN NEWS** has reported on dozens of important health campaigns by WHO and UNICEF, that have succeeded in mobilizing extensive resources, involving many different groups. What, then, has prevented both these agencies to deal with FGM and inspire the kind of initiatives they have successfully conducted in many other areas? These questions must be especially raised with their donors all over the world.

The Khartoum seminar of WHO was organized by the regional office in Alexandria, Egypt. WHO headquarters in Geneva had nothing to do with this except for sending a representative from their office of traditional medicine, Dr. Bannerman, a native of Ghana, who insisted that FGM should be introduced in hospitals in order to "preserve African tradition." He only backed down when it became clear that the seminar would fail unless he retracted his bid for medicalization. The recommendations of the seminar certainly were and are an important achievement and milestone paving the way for international and national action and prevention. (See **The HOSKEN REPORT** chapter on "WHO Seminar.")

But contrary to all expectations and hopes, nothing at all happened in the field as a result, and it took five years - until 1984 - for the Inter-African Committee to be organized at a NGO conference in Dakar sponsored by women's organizations.

Theoretically, with the discussions and publications of the WHO seminar, where I presented the introductory research paper on a global review of FGM and was a member of the secretariat, **WHO, UNICEF and all other governmental organizations and NGOs should have taken action to start prevention and education programs all over Africa.** Certainly this would have happened in every other case where international recommendations are made dealing with serious health problems. But since FGM affects women, the men who run all international agencies and programs in the health field obviously saw no reason to do anything at all.

UNICEF at first was reluctant to even accept the WHO recommendations, and its representatives in Africa continued to ignore them for years. I have yet to find a WHO office in Africa - which I visit every time I go to a country where FGM is practiced - that has heard about the WHO recommendations, let alone has taken action to implement them. The WHO representative neither attended nor sent anyone to the IAC training seminar in Ouagadougou, Burkina Faso, in July 1995, ignoring the IAC invitation.

WHO headquarters in Geneva failed to publicize or support the implementation of the 1979 Khartoum seminar recommendations and did not even inform their representatives, as I found out from my visits to WHO offices in Africa. The whole issue of FGM was forgotten and deliberately neglected. The Office of Family Health of WHO,* which is supposed to deal with FGM, continued to ignore it for many years much as they had always done before 1979, though the physicians who work there know all the facts.

Finally, two years ago, due to an inquiry by Senator Edward Kennedy and co-signed by two other senators, asking what WHO had accomplished regarding FGM since the 1979 Khartoum seminar, the WHO Family Health Office had to take note, as of course funding from the US is involved. WHO, much like all United Nations agencies, responds to one thing only: money. The Family Health Office clearly had problems to come up with anything in response to this inquiry, as they had done absolutely nothing about FGM; indeed WHO headquarters had only taken a marginal interest in the issue.

The lengthy response by WHO, of which I have a copy, could not conceal that the responsible people at WHO had completely ignored FGM and had not made the slightest attempt to promote or publicize the recommendations. **The response was accompanied by a one-page budget for $1 million, which WHO evidently asked for before even considering any action regarding FGM!** In concocting a response the WHO Family Health Office copied my statistics on the epidemiology of FGM and published them without even asking me, giving the names of two women I did not know on the credit line - Toubia and Sullivan. The Family Health Office, in answering my protest, claimed the printer got the credit mixed up. **But of course they know that this is a copyright violation and internationally classified as theft of intellectual property, which I also pointed out.**

This was evidently done to safeguard the funding by the US - money, rather than health, is clearly the most important concern for WHO. To conceal their failure, the WHO Family Health Office rushed into print everything they could get hold of, never mind who or what they violated, pretending they had done a great deal of research and work. Two months before the World Health Assembly met in Geneva, I received an urgent telephone call to send by express **The HOSKEN REPORT- Genital and Sexual Mutilation of Females.** At this occasion the Family Health Office held a briefing on FGM for the health ministries and published a large folder of papers on FGM, including much of my work without attribution. This publicity hoax was staged to assure funding, when in reality WHO had done nothing at all and had completely ignored the needs of women and FGM in Africa.

It is important for women to know that these international agencies use the most unscrupulous methods to preserve their prestige and acquire money. And for what? More paper work! Action in the field, where women desperately need help and health support, is utterly neglected by the bureaucrats, who rarely leave their offices in Geneva except to go to conferences. In Africa, and elsewhere in the field, WHO is totally ineffective, as the terrible conditions in maternity hospitals all over Africa demonstrate, lacking literally everything from equipment and tools to basic drugs and medicines, as I have seen for myself. **But of course the local WHO representatives never visit maternity hospitals. To talk to midwives, who handle all deliveries everywhere in Africa,** is below their dignity as physicians. They neither know nor care about women's health needs.

WHO claims to run a "Safe Motherhood Campaign," which now mainly consists of publishing a newsletter. Initially WHO paid some male physicians from Africa to write some research papers at Harvard Medical School. But the measures necessary to make childbirth safe have been known for many years, **though this takes real initiative in the field and hard work, both not available at WHO.**

---

*Division of Family Health, Dr. Tomris Turmen, Director; Dr. Mark Belsey, Program Manager; World Health Organization, CH-1211 Geneva 27, Switzerland.

In Africa, WHO has done nothing to improve childbirth services, as I saw again this past July in Burkina Faso, where I visited the maternity of the Yalgado Hospital, the main hospital in Ouagadougou. It still is located in the same bare building I first visited in 1977 which now serves twice as many women but has almost no equipment at all. And everywhere in Africa maternity hospitals and maternity services are neglected most of all and ignored, especially by WHO.

Women worldwide must understand what has been concealed and buried by empty propaganda and paperwork and useless research. **Women are not served by any of these international health agencies run by men and for the benefit of this male-dominated bureaucracy.** It is the male staff who gain from these international organizations which do not now and never have served the majority: women and children.

FGM has been stonewalled by sexual politics. Nothing else shows up the critical deficiencies as much and, worse, the deliberate neglect and malpractice by the men who run these international health bodies. They serve themselves and enhance their income and prestige. The devastating conclusion I have had to reach is: they simply do not care. These men claim to be physicians and concerned about health, but women and girls do not count because we do not add to their income or prestige. These male health professionals cannot be bothered to even pay attention to the needs of women, and this in an organization that is responsible for the health of the world.

Women must demand change; women everywhere must be heard and, if necessary, set up their own organizations to stop all the terrible waste and the callous disregard of real needs and the lying and posturing that goes on among the men who run all the international agencies while only seeking prestige and recognition for themselves.

The final example of mismanagement and lack of concern was the publication last year by WHO of the Briefing Papers on FGM - a publicity stunt geared to impress their sources for money. After appropriating my research and copying all the work on FGM they could gather - pretending WHO had something to do with it, which is completely untrue - **they forgot one critical concern: the medicalization of FGM!**

Only after I wrote repeatedly to the Family Health Office, pointing out this critical omission of failing to speak against the medicalization of FGM in the Briefing Papers, did that office produce and add another piece of paper citing their own forgotten resolution of 1982, which I had sent them. But the damage had been done: by their silence WHO was supporting medicalization. **The immediate result of this appalling omission is already visible in Egypt, where the health ministry - as cited above - is now introducing FGM into government hospitals** and at least one prominent physician at Cairo University has offered to run training programs for young physicians on how to mutilate female children. This would have not happened if WHO had officially opposed medicalization at their annual meeting in Geneva, as WHO enjoys great influence and prestige all over Africa and the Middle East.

It is interesting to note that WHO has not been heard from regarding this Egyptian affair nor did WHO do anything two years ago when in the Netherlands it was suggested that the daughters of Somalian immigrants might be mutilated in the hospitals at government expense to conform to Somali customs. **Medicalization is not only a violation of medical ethics, but it is a criminal violation of human rights.**

UNICEF, in turn, in 1980 sent out a policy paper on FGM to all field offices encouraging action and support for local groups working on eradication. This, after I gave a presentation at UNICEF headquarters on my research in Africa. But policies made in New York at headquarters have little influence in the field where each representative decides what to do. Most UNICEF representatives continue to be men.

To sum up, UNICEF has done almost nothing in the field in Africa over the years and there is no real policy at present. Lately, however, more women are working in UNICEF offices in Africa. The just-appointed executive director of UNICEF is a woman, Carol Bellamy, who headed the Peace Corps. At this writing, no changes in policy have been announced where FGM is concerned. James Grant, who ran UNICEF for nearly 20 years, totally ignored FGM and only a tiny fraction of the UNICEF budget was apportioned for this issue.

As this brief account documents, the international politics of FGM are certainly disastrous for women and girls. Prevention is much easier to organize than aggressive action against disease. There really is no excuse left for international agencies not to initiate prevention, especially since almost everywhere in Africa the issue is out in the open and discussed. More and more people want and ask for change, as my own experience with the **Childbirth Picture Books** demonstrates (see Appendix). The training seminar* in Burkina Faso certainly documented great readiness for change as the participants from 22 countries all confirmed. **The issue now is how to implement change quickly and effectively.**

But funding to date has been completely inadequate, and given the economic problems in Africa every action has to be supported by funds from abroad. It is no longer a question of if FGM will be eradicated, but when.

As long as men are in charge of all international development health and population programs the issue will not be given the priority that is needed. **What is necessary is to make preventive action part of every education and training program, every initiative and action, all development, health and population programs on every level and everywhere.**

CONCLUSION

The facts documented here from direct experience over many years show that the politics of FGM are sexual politics, first and most of all. The questions that must be raised are: where are the men, and where are, first of all, the African leaders to convince their brothers that FGM must be stopped if African countries are to effectively participate in development and pull themselves out of their continuously deteriorating economic morass, the escalating violence, the tribal and ethnic warfare which is increasingly engulfing more and more of this continent.

But where are the international leaders? Where are the professionals who claim to guide international political life? Most of all, where are the men who for years have been concerned with population policies that are so vital to the future of our world? Why have none of them ever spoken up and demanded that the mutilation of helpless children must stop? **Not a single leader in Africa has set an example with his own family, proclaiming publicly that the daughters of his family will not be mutilated and that the family's sons will not take a mutilated bride. And that is what needs to be done to set an example.**

Where are the men who claim the leadership of international institutions and the world? Why has no one in government or in the private sector spoken up and condemned these damaging practices? **Is it too much to ask that these men who work internationally and who have excluded women from leadership, to finally show some courage and speak up to demand that this useless butchery be stopped?** How can we respect men who lack the initiative and courage to see that this senseless attack on the genitalia of their own daughters be stopped wherever it goes on? How can we trust men such as the leaders of WHO, UNICEF and USAID who still refuse to deal with FGM in realistic ways by providing the necessary resources to do so effectively?

It is a shocking indictment of the sexual politics of men that even today, after more than 15 years of international discussion of FGM, not one of the many leaders who claim to have power in Africa and internationally has spoken up asking that men everywhere come together to publicly condemn FGM and jointly organize a campaign by and for men to stop these terrible mutilations of girls.

FGM is not a private matter; it is a public concern and an international crime that must be condemned by all leaders who claim our attention and following. The secrecy has been removed once and for all. How can women respect leaders too cowardly to speak up among their peers for other men to join them in stopping the needless torture of female children? **The silence by men condones and supports the continuation of FGM.** Women everywhere need to know that this is what really is going on today. To date, not a single man anywhere has had the courage to speak up, least of all in Africa.

---

*Inter-African Committee Regional Training Seminar, July 17-21, 1995, Ouagadougou, Burkina Faso.

WOMEN SPEAK ABOUT THEIR LIVES

According to long-held traditions women are supposed to be silent and obey: these patriarchal family rules and customs still prevail in much of the world. The more traditional the society the stronger the rules are enforced. It is the male head of the family who speaks for women. Female family members are never asked for their opinions; they follow orders and remain mute, because if they don't, violence is used to enforce these patriarchal rules. This is the way it has always been all over the world. Old women are often enlisted by flattery and designated as "keepers of tradition."

Silence has protected the system of male rule and privilege enforced by male violence which has continued for centuries all over the world, as all historic texts confirm.

But recently, after this hierarchical family system of unquestioned male rule has continued as long as anyone can remember and literally everywhere, women have begun to speak. **This revolutionary change is still very new and sometimes hesitant, but gradually all over the world women are speaking ever louder, they are telling their stories and demanding change. Women have begun to speak for themselves!** Women are finding their voices: "We shall no longer be silent and submit to male violence, we shall no longer be coerced, mutilated, raped and exploited as male property. We shall be heard everywhere, make our own decisions, and control our own bodies and lives!"

Women everywhere in the world are revolting against the conspiracy of silence in order to break patriarchal domination and violence: **the dreadful truth about male violence against women and children of their own families, their wives, mothers and daughters, is coming out in the open everywhere in the world.** It is being discussed, documented and recorded.*

Women's words are being heard. More and more women are finding the courage by supporting each other to stand up and demand change, to demand justice and their rights. Of course, patriarchal reaction has been swift, enlisting the male-dominated media in an evil alliance of fundamentalists of every stripe, supported by patriarchal religions led by Islam, Roman Catholicism and the "reborn Christian" politicians of the U.S.

But once the seeds of freedom have been sown on such long-deprived fertile ground they will grow. There is no stopping them: women everywhere are joining as communication is reaching all areas of our one world. We are speaking for ourselves, often for the first time, and we are demanding to be heard everywhere - Asia, Africa and the Middle East, in Europe and the Americas, in the Pacific and Australia. The issues are the same. **Women are speaking in all different languages, telling their own stories and demanding to be heard. Most of all we want justice, we demand change and abolishment of the patriarchal order, and recognition of our human rights.**

We are going to make the decisions that affect our lives and our children's as well as the world which our labor has built. And we shall speak up for what is right in each family. It is the family where boys first learn violence and girls are forced to submit, where the male family head imposes his rule by violence and boys learn from his example, where violence is taught as the order of the day. **And this must change first, because it is in the family where our children are socialized, where their lives and values are formed.**

Women from all continents and countries are speaking about the injustices they suffer, their deprivation, beatings, rape and fear of male violence - which have been covered up by silence for centuries. NO MORE! From all over the world it is the same terrible story - but at last the silence has been broken, and this is the first step towards real change.

---

* **The Country Reports on Human Rights Practices,** published annually by the US Department of State and submitted to Congress by law, have reported on human rights violations around the world for many years. Family violence against women has been included for the past 10 or more years, documenting that in all countries around the world (193 in 1993 and 1994) male violence against female family members persists. Female Genital Mutilation is also reported in all countries where this practice exists.

More and more women in Africa are speaking up against the violence of female genital mutilation (FGM) in their families, sanctioned by their patriarchal communities in this war-torn continent. They are from the most diverse regions of Africa and the Middle East with very different living conditions: but the **girls and women subjected to these tortures suffer the same agonizing pain, the same debilitating health damage, and the same deep psychological wounds**. And everywhere these human rights violations are tolerated by the rest of the world in the name of "culture," which is still used as an excuse to turn away.

Many millions are spent on development and population programs that protect "culture" instead of protecting the health and lives of girls and women who suffer the harrowing violence of the operation. The horrifying experience of the wedding night, when often as very young girls they are brutalized by a man they barely know who has bought their bodies to bear his children, is followed by the prolonged ordeal of childbirth from which many women never recover. Sexual intercourse often becomes a torturous experience of repeated pain from which women are unable to escape.

The reality of these traditional practices has never been discussed from a woman's view. Anthropologists claim that this is "culture" and therefore a treasure to preserve - no matter how many girls and women are tortured to death. **The patriarchal system is quite international and globally protected**. Where are the men today speaking for change?

Most African women continue to live in rural areas and are charged with feeding their many children from what they grow themselves, after enduring the excruciatingly painful births due to their mutilated bodies. Carrying water, growing and preparing the food with the most primitive tools, takes many hours every day of exhausting work. Why add to the burdens of subsistence farming and its hundreds of exhausting daily tasks by mutilating women's bodies, which clearly saps their strength and has permanent damaging effects?

The rituals, the myths, and often also the age at which girls are mutilated vary from region to region, with many different rites and beliefs. But the basic reason is the same, though rarely pronounced: **the mutilations are done even now because men require them -** because they guarantee male domination and control. An African man will not spend the brideprice to purchase a girl who is not excised or infibulated, according to the local requirement. In traditional village societies the father seeks to get a good price for his daughters, and a girl who is not suitably initiated - that is, mutilated as local custom demands - is not acceptable to a husband and his family. Therefore every father has a financial incentive to see to it that his daughters are mutilated according to local tradition.

All family decisions in Africa are made by men. Women do not have the means to pay for the operations, which by local standards are a costly affair. **In traditional African societies women own nothing, not the land they till nor their homes, and what a woman earns belongs to her husband**. Women carry out the mutilations for which they are highly rewarded: it is one of the few paid occupations for women in traditional Africa. But even there, the men who circumcise the boys get paid more. In most of Africa FGM is an all-female affair, especially in Moslem areas. **But the responsibility for the mutilations rests with men, because men make FGM a requirement for marriage. And marriage is the only career for every woman - even now there is no alternative.**

Men frequently claim they have nothing to do with FGM, which means they are not doing the actual cutting. But as in all important family matters, men alone make the decisions, and men everywhere control the purse strings.

Most women in rural areas are still illiterate - for instance, in francophone Africa, in rural areas, often more than 90 percent cannot read or write. **Women have to carry out the decisions made by men regarding the rural household - as women, according to tradition, cannot own land.** When a man dies, his land and all his possessions are taken by his male relatives; the children are kept as part of the agricultural labor force on their father's land controlled by his family, and the widow is sent back to her family with nothing.

A wife, according to African traditions, has no rights of her own, she is the property of men. Community decisions are made by the male village elders, women are never consulted at all. A man often buys a second or third wife from the money he made selling the produce his women grew - and installs his new wife in his house, without questions.

In the rapidly growing urban areas, the situation of women is often even worse as they have no land to grow food for their children and no way to earn any money to buy food. But for the most part, men only go to town, leaving their wives and children behind. They claim to go to town to earn some money, but there are few jobs for the unskilled, and in every African town one can see clusters of men hanging around, often drinking and accosting everyone who comes along.

The women and children are left behind in the countryside to fend for themselves. The men come home to the village when they please, to eat the food the women grow for their children and to father another child. Often they also infect women with sexually transmitted diseases or AIDS, which they have acquired in town. The men decide what their wives must grow on their land, when their daughters are to be excised and to whom they should be married. They negotiate the brideprice, take the money and go back to town. Men often spend long periods away from home, and many have another wife in town while the rural women are left alone to support the entire household from their work.

Men in Africa have no legal or other obligation to support their children - that is the traditional task of women. According to tradition, children in rural areas join the agricultural labor force as soon as they are able to work - girls have to take care of the younger children while the women work in the fields. If there are schools in the area, boys are sent, the girls are needed for housework; the school fees are too high to send both.

In Moslem societies men have to support their families - so religion prescribes. But in reality they always can get a divorce, which frees them from all obligations of maintenance after three months. As the records show, divorce is very frequent in Moslem Africa. Many influential men have dozens of wives, though only four at any one time.

This is the general background and family context of the stories the women relate. These personal accounts are from all different areas of Africa, yet it is astonishing how great the similarity of the oppression women suffer and the appalling violence practiced by men everywhere - without the slightest compassion - often against their own children and all female members of their families. As my many visits to Africa confirm, as well as interviews with African leaders and United Nations delegates, the same patriarchal system prevails throughout and to the highest levels of African leadership.

The women whose stories are related here, to be sure, are the exceptions as they are able to tell about their lives. They have succeeded in getting an education, which makes it possible for them to speak about their own experiences from a critical view, evaluating what they have suffered as persons in their own right and demanding change for their children. They represent only a tiny minority of women in Africa today. Most women are still illiterate and therefore have limited means of communication. They do not know that any other way of life is possible, so they have no choice but to cope with the degradation and male violence that is their daily life, trying to protect their children as best they can.

SOMALIA

In Somalia, where more than 98 percent of the population is Moslem, initiation, to which traditionally all female children are subjected, takes place in the home among women of the neighborhood. The operation is performed without ceremony, much like castrating an animal. Fatuma tells her story:

> "I was forcibly held down after the women stripped me. I had been asleep when they came at dawn. I was barely 6 years old and terrified; I did not know what was happening. They pulled my legs apart and held them open. A big old woman sat down facing me and started to cut me with a large knife . . . it hurt terribly. I tried to free myself and screamed and screamed . . . the last thing I remember was blood all over, spurting from between my legs. Then I passed out . . . "

Fatuma has lived in England for some time. She is one of the very few Somali women from an influential family who could afford to have the terrible mutilation, inflicted on her as a child, partially repaired at a private clinic in London. But no one can restore the clitoris that was removed, together with most of the nerve endings in this most sensitive area of her body. **Cutting out this organ is the purpose of the operation, which is still performed annually on hundreds of thousands of helpless female children.** Fatuma continues:

"But that is not all . . . In Somalia, for a girl to be able to get married - and that is her only purpose in life - she must be closed. Her virginity must be visibly proven. She is inspected by the female relatives of the man who pays the bride price for her.

After the clitoris is cut out, as well as some of the surrounding flesh, the sides of the large lips are scraped or sliced and then sewn together with catgut, or most of the time they are just fastened together with some thorns. Then the legs are tied together and the girl must remain motionless until the wound heals, closing the vagina except for a tiny opening to pass urine and later menstrual blood."

Thus virginity is guaranteed and this fetches a high brideprice for the father.

"The days after the operation were terrible; the pain when I had to urinate went on for months; and later, each menstruation was an ordeal.

I was lucky at that. I guess because I bled so much the wound was not too badly infected. All the women examine the bleeding hole with their fingers to make sure that everything has been completely cut out. I had fainted from the pain, but I saw them operate on my little sister a few years later. I tried to warn her, but there was nothing I could do.

My sister was very ill for many months, and she has never been the same since. All her carefree laughter was gone. Worst of all, she is unable to have children, so her husband took another wife. Fortunately, he did not divorce her which would be a terrible disgrace for the whole family."

The grandmothers, who take charge of the younger women of the family, insist on the operations. All women believe that the operation is essential; without it, a girl is "lost." No man would ever marry her. Men demand a closed bride; the smaller the opening, the higher the brideprice. Virginity is tied to the honor of the patriarchal family. A girl belongs to her father, a woman to her husband - a female has no right to her own body or life.

Fatuma, who has somehow learned to live with her fate, is an exception; but then, she lives abroad. She patiently continued to answer my questions:

"In Somalia, when the wedding takes place, it is necessary for the bride to be cut open, because no man can penetrate the artificial barrier. Some men use their own knives - but since they don't know anatomy the results are often devastating. Most of the men ask a midwife to cut their bride - lately also physicians are used. Intercourse takes place at once, and frequently, to keep the wound from closing again. The bloody sheets are shown to the neighbors, demonstrating that the bridegroom got a closed bride."

Fatuma had the operation to open her done under anesthesia at a clinic. But the young brides of Somalia are not that lucky. **The wedding night is a traumatic experience and the following days a prolonged ordeal.** All intercourse frequently means recurring pain, but to have children is all-important for every woman: only through childbirth can a woman gain some security.

Divorce is frequent, especially in the polygamous households of the well-to-do men. A divorced wife goes back to her parents, and often some of the brideprice has to be paid back - depending on the length of the marriage and whether any children resulted, who are the property of the husband. All these arrangements are commercial transactions between men in cash or in kind - trading a woman for camels or cash or other goods.

Once back with her family of origin, the divorced wife is re-infibulated and then another marriage is negotiated by the father; generally the second time she is sold for a lesser brideprice. A European physician who worked in Somalia kept a record of the many marriages of his patients, who were from well-off families as only the well-to-do can afford to consult a physician. The trade in women that he recorded is quite remarkable. Women often marry a number of times. Each marriage involves a financial transaction in cash or in kind by the father and lengthy negotiations between the men of the families. The women are never consulted at all.

Occasionally, however, so the doctor recorded, a new wife left the husband's household if she did not get on with the other wives. Some of the women entered and left four or five marriages in the space of a few years, with or without children. Often second, third, or fourth wives joined or left a variety of different households of men of means, as poor men cannot afford to purchase several wives.

An astonishing family structure emerges based on the trade in women by the wealthier men, who often buy 10 or more wives in succession, though religion says they cannot have more than four at any one time. The older ones are divorced and replaced with young and fertile ones to build large families, which means power in traditional societies. Some of the women leaders I met in Mogadishu lived with their extended families in large compounds behind high walls, with many women and their children sharing a series of buildings surrounding an open yard. Apparently each compound housed the family of just one man.

A few years before the drought, the civil war and collapse of the Somalian Government led by Siad Barre, a national campaign to eradicate FGM was started. This campaign was led by the Somali Women's Democratic Organization (SWDO) jointly with the Italian Association for Women in Development (AIDoS). This remarkable initiative is described and documented in **The HOSKEN REPORT** as well as in **WIN NEWS.** This unprecedented campaign was a unique achievement in Africa and provides an important example and guidelines in form of the education programs which were developed. Somalia now has no government: all law and order have collapsed and violence rules the day.

In June 1988, this campaign organized an international conference in order to attract world attention and support. This historic meeting was held in the Great Hall of the Parliament, decorated by a huge fresco of a Somalian woman reaching to the sky with her outstretched hands followed by a large crowd of Somalian people whom she leads. This conference focused on the national education and information campaign seeking guidance and ideas from participants from other African countries where similar campaigns are underway. Educational materials and initiatives had been prepared for every sector of Somalian society and government. **Training activities had been started by both women and men delivering the message that FGM must be stopped** because it does irreparable harm to the whole society, which must be freed of such traditional impediments to development.

It is astonishing that the international press, including all US television programs which covered Somalia daily and reported live from all over the country for more than a year about the famine and civil war, failed to report anything at all about this campaign. What is more, **they entirely ignored the facts that every Somalian woman is infibulated and the social and economic damage that result from these mutilations** or that the leadership had begun to reject FGM by supporting a national effort to educate their own people.

This discriminatory reporting by US media in particular, and international media in general, all controlled by men, is doing enormous damage to developing countries and women everywhere. It is this media bias which women must challenge. **Women-owned media, including WIN NEWS, which reports by, for and about women all over the world, are trying to correct such damaging omissions.**

Somalian society, which tried too late to free itself of its violent family traditions, is now paying the terrible price by the total collapse of law and order. **Violence is learned in each family where young boys are initiated by the extreme brutality of family customs** to which all girls - their own sisters - are subjected. Usually the mutilations are performed on girls at the age of 5 to 7 - recently even younger. Boys witness the torture of their sisters which is accepted as normal treatment of all females.

Men who learn such extreme violence in childhood do not hesitate to use force against women, as could be observed on all TV broadcasts from that country during the famine. Somalian boys and young men were shown brandishing weapons and hoarding food - which meant power - while their sisters and mothers were left to starve. **Violence still rules that society and the same can be observed elsewhere in Africa** where civil wars of extreme brutality are the order of the day, victimizing women and children most of all.

The traditions of mutilating female children as family custom have a permanent effect on the whole society and that must be recognized. More and more areas of Africa are beset by constant civil wars: in many of these regions traditional practices of extreme violence and brutality against girls and women are accepted family customs.

Modern weapons were introduced in these traditional societies by their male leaders to rule the population by force. They are now destroying more and more African countries and societies. For many African men, brought up with family traditions of violent abuse of female children and women and all who cannot defend themselves, **brutal force is the accepted road to power and success.**

African leadership should look to their women, who are now beginning to speak up everywhere and demanding that the violent traditions must stop. The all-male African governments must be persuaded to listen to the women in their own societies and ask for their advice and help to change the violent family traditions which are at the root of all the ethnic violence, destroying more and more African societies and countries.

SUDAN

In no other country of Africa have there been as many efforts and initiatives over the past 50 years to eradicate infibulation, which continues to be the mutilation preferred by most men throughout Moslem northern Sudan. The South, where civil war has raged for decades, is inhabited by very different ethnic groups who have never practiced any form of female mutilations, though due to intermarriage infibulation is beginning to spread there. However, in the twin cities of Khartoum and Omdurman the practice has prevailed for as long as anyone can remember.

A young woman in her late 20's, still unmarried and living with her parents in Khartoum, tells her story:

> "I was infibulated first when I was 5 years old. I remember every bit of it still - the terrible pain and lying tied up for several weeks. It hurt so much that I cried and cried. I could not understand why this was done to me.
>
> When I was nearly 12, my aunts one day examined me. They declared that I was not closed enough. They took me to the midwife who lives a few streets away. When I noticed where they were taking me, I tried to run away; but they held me tight and dragged me into the midwife's house. I screamed for help and tried to free myself; but I was not strong.
>
> They held me down and they put a cover over my mouth so I could not scream. Then the midwife cut me again; and this time, the woman who operated on me made sure that I was closed.
>
> They carried me home. The pain was terrible. My legs were tied together and I could not move. I could not urinate, and my stomach became all swollen. I was terribly hot one moment, then shaking with cold. This was during the dry season of the sandstorms, when it is hard to breathe. I don't know how many days I was lying there. Then the midwife came again. I screamed as hard as I could, as I thought she was going to cut me again. Then I lost consciousness.
>
> I woke up in a hospital ward. There were moaning women all around me. I was terrified; I did not know where I was. I was in terrible pain; my legs and my genital area were terribly swollen and I hurt all over.
>
> Later I was told that the infibulation had been cut open to let the urine and the puss out. I was too weak to even cry; I did not care anymore. I wanted to die. Why would my mother do this to me? What had I done to be so terribly hurt?
>
> It is years later now. The doctors told me that I could never have children because of the infection which continues to cause me pain. Therefore, no one will marry me; no one wants a wife who cannot have a child. I do not want to get married because I am afraid that I shall be hurt again. I sit at home alone and cry a lot. I look at my mother and at my aunts, and I ask them: 'Why did you do this terrible thing to me?'"

Though there have been continuous efforts in Sudan by many committed people for more than two generations to stop infibulation, this most drastic form of mutilation continues to be practiced throughout northern Sudan, including in all urban areas.

In **The HOSKEN REPORT** chapter on Sudan, the facts and the historic background are documented. The Inter-African Committee affiliate of Sudan is now headed by Amna Abdel Rahman Hassan,* who energetically leads this initiative to eradicate the mutilations. But it appears that the male Moslem leadership of Sudan has other priorities than to stop the infibulation of their women, and this is the way it has always been in this very traditional Moslem society.

In Sudan, which has a long-established medical school started by the British during colonial times as well as the oldest midwifery training system in Africa, first developed more than 50 years ago by two British Army nurses, more initiatives to eradicate FGM have been organized than anywhere else. Sudanese physicians have been in the leadership to eradicate these mutilations.

The most comprehensive clinical study on FGM ever made, published in the Sudan Medical Journal, was by **Dr. Ahmed Abu El Futuh Shandall, Circumcision and Infibulation of Females: A General Consideration of the Problems and a Clinical Study of the Complications in Sudanese Women.** It was based on the case histories of more than 3,000 women who were patients at Khartoum City Hospital over a 10-year period. This study provided detailed tabulation of the terrible effects of FGM on women's health. **Dr. Asma El Dareer,** in her book **Woman, Why Do You Weep? - Circumcision and Its Consequences,** conducted a unique survey and opinion poll of women and men to determine the extent of the operations in a large part of the country as well as the ideas of the people regarding the practice. It found that men overwhelmingly support the continuation of FGM.

Many people, including physicians and midwives, take advantage of this male support for FGM and carry on a lucrative trade performing the mutilations in "sanitary" ways. **This modernization and medicalization of FGM must be strenuously opposed.** The transfer of a damaging traditional practice into a paid medical intervention in a modern hospital or clinic is a dangerous development, as greedy physicians will promote the mutilations everywhere. FGM is an effective way for men to control women psychologically as well as their sexuality. Influential African men who support medicalization, claiming "to make it safe," are encouraged by many physicians who stand to make a lot of money from the operations, as is already happening in Sudan and Egypt and other countries as well.

It was amazing to read in a booklet on FGM by Nahid Toubia, a Sudanese expatriate living in the US who practiced medicine in Khartoum, that she believes FGM is like breast implants. **To compare the torturous genital mutilations inflicted on little girls by force with an elective operation of adult women in modern operating rooms,** demonstrates an astonishing lack of compassion. She also argued this point on a national television program in the US, before an audience that had no information of the conditions under which most African and Sudanese girls are mutilated. To claim that little girls undergo the mutilations by choice is a gross distortion of the facts. Toubia saw plenty of mutilations in Sudan forced on helpless little girls who do not understand why they are tortured nor about the terrible results. **FGM is prohibited by child abuse laws in Europe and in all countries where such laws exist; it is classified globally as human rights violation.**

Medicalization of FGM is increasing everywhere the practice exists, though of course in most African countries very few families can afford to have the mutilations done by professionals. In Khartoum and Cairo, this modernization of the practice is widespread in large towns as there are more physicians and trained health workers. The World Health Organization opposed the medicalization at the 1979 seminar in Khartoum on **"Traditional Practices Affecting the Health of Women and Children,"** though participants from the Khartoum University medical faculty supported it. But since then, WHO has been silent or ineffective in opposing medicalization, which is a violation of medical ethics, and this is very damaging. (See chapter on the Politics of FGM.)

*****Sudan National Committee on Traditional Practices Affecting the Health of Women and Children, P.O. Box 10418, Khartoum, Sudan.**

Here is the story of Nafisa, a middle-aged woman who lives in Omdurman and is from a very traditional family. Nafisa was married at 14. Penetration took 15 days, as her husband was too proud to ask a midwife to deinfibulate his bride. Every Sudanese man claims he accomplished this feat himself, no matter at what cost to his bride, though many secretly hire midwives. As for many other young women, intercourse for Nafisa continued to be very painful. She described how, at the birth of her first child, she was hung from the rafters with ropes under her arms "the traditional way," while the birth attendant squatted in front under her and cut her open when the infibulation scar began to tear.

Now Nafisa has five children, two of them girls. The first one was infibulated and nearly died from loss of blood. She had to be taken to the hospital and was ill for months, and is still weak. Her marriage had to be postponed. **The physicians warned the parents about infibulating the other daughter, who is terrified because of what happened to her sister.** Nafisa persuaded her husband not to have it done; to protect the child from family members, especially grandmothers, they decided to send her away to school.

This is what Zuraya, who is now 25, related about her and her sisters' mutilations. She was brought up in Europe where she and her family went to live:

"My sisters and I lived in Europe where we went to school. Then my two sisters, my mother and I went to visit our family in Sudan; we thought we were going for a holiday. We were not told that we were going to be infibulated. But the day before the operation was planned another girl next door was operated and she died. We were so afraid - we did not want to die. Our parents told us that this had to be done, it was an obligation and there was no other way.

We were taken to the excisor's house, we fought back as hard as we could, it was terrible; we thought we would be killed. The pain was terrible, there was no anesthetic. We were held down by some strong women, one held my mouth so I could not scream, the other held my chest and arms and another held my legs open so the midwife could cut. After they infibulated us ropes were tied around our legs and we were kept that way for what seemed an endless time. We had to try to pass water, no matter how terribly it hurt, because they said if you don't something is wrong and you have to be operated all over again. We were lucky, none of us died.

But the memory of the pain never goes away, and every time I have to go to the toilet I am reminded again. Luckily I was still very young when it was done. A friend of mine was infibulated in her teens, she suffers from nightmares and often wakes up screaming. She is very depressed. I shall never get married so I don't have to be re-opened and have the operation again. I cannot stand to even think of it."

This letter from Germany, by a Sudanese mother, was addressed to WIN NEWS:

"Dear Frau Hosken:

I heard of WIN from a friend. I am a Sudanese graduate in education from Munich. You cannot help me, but you can help other Sudanese women who, like me, have been through the hell of the pharaonic operation [infibulation]. This is done to make you feel nothing but pain when you make love . . .

I was closed after being cut when I was 10. The daya who did it closed me very tight. It was done when my mother was away, she is Egyptian and was only cut. In Sudan it is said the tighter the bride the more the husband will love her. When you are closed it is like you are in prison in yourself.

In Germany I heard from the other students about the pleasure of love. There is no feeling left when I touch myself, in this way it is made sure you are a virgin.

I have been married for three years and I have a daughter. My aunts want her to be cut and closed like they are. My husband says the Turkish doctors here in Germany would do it without pain, it costs 1,000 DM and if done before 2 the child will not remember. My husband says it has to be done or no one will marry her.

Why can't women be left with our bodies how we are born? In a few weeks my child who is 2 will be operated - this is better than what I suffered. I don't give my name but please write to other women about our suffering . . ."

From a gynecologist practicing in Khartoum and teaching at the medical school:

"Of course I am opposed to excision and especially infibulation. I see the terrible results in the hospital every day. I try to persuade all my patients and especially their husbands to stop these terrible practices. But you asked me about my family: that is a difficult question. Obviously, I reject having my daughters operated. But in my community here in Khartoum a girl could never find a husband unless she is operated. All the leading families do it, also those connected with the university. Girls who are not, are excluded from social life.

So I solved this problem in this way: my wife and I went through all the preparations for the traditional celebration and invited our families and friends. The traditional excisor whom we hired was instructed to only pretend to do the operation, which is now done in a room and not before the guests in the yard as in the past. The excisor was well paid for her compliance and her silence. Our daughters were given a whiff of ether so they did not know what was done, as girls at that age can't keep secrets. They believed they had been operated. That is the only way we could protect them when they were children. Of course when they were older we told them."

But that physicians and community leaders should work together and set an example with their own families never occurred to this leader of medicine in Khartoum.

A young Sudanese medical school student at the University of Khartoum relates:

"I have undergone complete excision - that is, my clitoris and labia minora were cut out when I was seven. Fortunately I was not infibulated. I remember every detail of this terrible ordeal and the days of suffering that followed which at the time I managed to bear as I was told that I had to be excised to become a real woman and get married. It was said that without the operation girls are unclean and all men would reject them. Of course I believed what I was told - I had no way to learn the truth. I had heard all kinds of stories from my girl friends.

Early one morning, I was still asleep, I was taken from my bed and carried to the backyard where a group of women were ready for me. They held me down and opened my legs. The operator with a razor blade set to work immediately, and before I could even cry out blood was spurting all over my legs and a terrible pain pierced me through and through. I had never felt such an overwhelming sensation and lost consciousness.

I continued to bleed for some days. My mother and her sisters got very worried; I could not even raise my head. After some days, I slowly began to regain some strength to drink and eat a little. But when I had to urinate the unbearable searing pain returned. Slowly the wound healed and I was very happy that now I was pure and clean and would become a real woman. Of course by now I know that these are all myths, and I was made to suffer this terrible ordeal for nothing. Worse, the operation would most likely cause terrible problems if and when I have children.

I don't know that I want to get married at all. I have no interest in the male students I work with in medical school. I can't imagine allowing a man to touch me, let alone have sexual intercourse; the very idea I found revolting when I first learned about it in medical school. I still live with my family, I have no alternative. In our society a woman cannot live alone or share a house with other female students.

Every day I pass the place in the yard where I was excised more than 20 years ago - and my younger sisters after me; I still hear their cries, and their wailing went on for days. I could not help them at the time. But this is why I insisted on studying medicine. I don't know what I shall be able to do as everyone still believes in the operations, they are going on all the time, all my friends are excised or infibulated.

The wealthy people now go to doctors to have their daughters done; there are many private clinics, and the people who do the operations become rich - even women physicians now do it. I am determined to find a way to stop it. Soon I shall have my medical degree, but that is only the first step. Of course I know that here in Sudan many previous attempts to stop the mutilations have failed even in the city of Khartoum. But I am determined to succeed even if it takes the rest of my life. . ."

The 1979 WHO seminar, cited above, was a groundbreaking event for all of Africa and especially Sudan, which acted as host country. The seminar opened international discussion of FGM including for international nongovernmental organizations (NGOs) working in health and development, which up to then claimed that they could not work on prevention because FGM was a forbidden subject on cultural grounds.

The seminar once more stimulated professional and medical discussion in Sudan but no major actions resulted, though the medical and midwifery schools and many other organizations were and are teaching to stop FGM. All these efforts are documented in the chapter on Sudan of **The HOSKEN REPORT**.

But given the ongoing civil war in the South and the political problems, there are few resources available to educate women and improve their status, though many young women study medicine at the university in Khartoum. **Family decisions are strongly influenced by tradition; men make all decisions in the polygamous patriarchal families.**

EGYPT

According to medical researchers, FGM has been practiced in Egypt for more than 2,000 years. It is claimed that archeologists discovered that some female mummies they had found had been excised. In **The HOSKEN REPORT, the "Case History of Egypt" and the chapter on the history of FGM provide extensive research and documentation.** Though it is not officially admitted, it is estimated that the vast majority of young girls in Egypt continue to be excised even in urban areas; among the older generation almost all women are mutilated. In southern Egypt and on the border of Sudan, infibulation prevails.

It is astonishing that though many leaders of the medical profession claim to be opposed to FGM, many private clinics do the operations for a fee. While there is a statute that prohibits dayas, the traditional midwives, from doing the operations, there is no prohibition for medical practitioners. **The Cairo Family Planning Association, a private group that pioneered family planning in Egypt under the leadership of Aziza Hussein, initiated the very first program to teach against FGM in the early 1980's.** They now have more than 12 years of experience in the field and recently affiliated with the Inter-African Committee. Their groundbreaking activities are described in **The HOSKEN REPORT**, and their annual reports, which cover their educational activities and campaigns, are reported in **WIN NEWS**. Workshops and meetings held all over Cairo as well as with village and religious leaders, teachers, social workers, health professionals and physicians, are detailed in these reports, which provide some excellent guidelines for prevention.

The extent of the involvement of medical professionals was reported at 20 percent by the Cairo Family Planning Association in 1991, up from 15 percent in 1986. **At the International Conference on Population and Development, in September 1994, FGM was widely discussed.** The Cairo Family Planning Association held an internationally reported meeting showing that, on average, some 80 percent of girls and women are mutilated. After President Hosni Mubarak of Egypt, in an interview shown on CNN, claimed FGM was not practiced in Egypt, CNN showed an actual operation of an 8-year-old girl which had been videotaped the day before in an apartment in Cairo. This created an uproar, and resulted in a statement that legislation against FGM would be considered. Instead, several months after the conference, a leading gynecologist at Cairo University proposed to the Government to start training physicians on how to mutilate girls the medical way.

An Egyptian physician strongly opposed to FGM talked to women patients about their operations. They all stated that they were assaulted, chased, held down, immobilized and mutilated by force. They were never asked, and were deceived about the procedure:

> "They attacked me by surprise - I saw the daya holding a razor, then she cut me." // "I was shocked, I did not comprehend what was happening to me or why, I screamed for help but no one helped me." // "It was terrible, I could not understand why I was being held down or by whom, I screamed until they put a rag over my mouth - then I saw my aunt laughing at me." // "I could not believe my mother was with them, they all attacked me early one morning while I was still sleeping, I could not defend myself." // "I cried as loud as I could: Why are you doing this to me? I was terrified and could not understand why I was being attacked or why my parents would hurt me so terribly. I cried for days. I never trusted my mother again."

Mona is a 23-year-old graduate of a commercial school and a Copt. She is single and works as a secretary in a college in Cairo. Mona was operated on at the age of 9:

"My mother had nothing at all to do with the whole process. . . It was a decision between my father and his sister. My aunt told me that she was taking me on an outing when I realized that we were going to the doctor's clinic. . .

My aunt and the young Moslem doctor and his male assistant caught hold of me. The doctor explained that this was necessary for my future, to guarantee my marriage. They held me tight and I couldn't run away. The male assistant stretched my legs apart, and the doctor cut off the tip of my clitoris with his scissors. . .

My aunt carried me to her home which was close to the doctor's clinic and I spent the rest of the day in bed. For seven days she gave me chicken to eat and insisted on taking care of the wound. The doctor came to see me four days after the operation and declared that everything was all right. My aunt followed the same procedure with my cousins, as well as my three sisters.

The people around me still explain that circumcision is as important as keeping clean and is necessary for marriage. The dayas emphasize the importance of the operation, and claim that what is cut off is ugly and the husband would not experience any pleasure if it is not cut off. All girls I know are circumcised."

Most of the operations are done by dayas, but barbers are also traditionally involved in both male and female operations. They make a lot of money from the mutilations, and so do physicians who perform the operations on the daughters of wealthy families.

A young woman physician who was expecting a baby was asked about the operation, as she had been excised herself as a child. Her answer raises serious doubts about the medical education provided at Egyptian universities. **The young woman stated that if her baby should be a girl she would circumcise her herself,** as some doctors in Cairo were reluctant to do the operation. She claimed it was important to do the operation for three main reasons: the first one was religion - she was a Moslem (though in Egypt it is also done by all Christian Copts). The second reason she cited was aesthetic and cosmetic - she wished to remove something ugly, disfiguring and repulsive, to make the girl more attractive to her future husband when the time came to get married. And finally, she claimed this would protect the girl from sexual stimulation which could damage her life. Of course, tradition was also important, she stated, and then she claimed that husbands preferred their wives to be excised.

Here is the story of Leila, an Egyptian Moslem woman, who lives in Greater Cairo with her husband. Leila was raised in Cairo and went to school before she was married. She was less than 9 years old when she and her two sisters were operated on together:

"My grandmother and my father decided that I should be circumcised according to custom and tradition. A daya came and performed the operation at home. I didn't know about it, except on the day itself, when my grandmother told me it was necessary. I was very afraid, especially when the woman came, opened her bag, and took out the razor and the disinfectant. I screamed from pain, and my grandmother and my aunt, who were with me, were greatly concerned.

It took more than one week before I was able to resume my usual activities. I was made to sit in warm water and disinfectant twice a day. . .

There was no special celebration after the operation; but for a week, I was given special food such as chicken and meat and sweets.

Now when I wash myself and touch myself, there is nothing there; and I don't feel anything. The daya cut off the clitoris and the two leaves. It has to be done or you can't get married, I was told at the time. I never have discussed it with my husband.

Recently I began to ask my friends about the operations. Most of them were operated when they were young, mostly under 10. Some claim it is necessary to be clean; but I don't know. I also learned there are accidents; I guess I was lucky, though the pain was terrible. But I don't think I shall have it done on my daughters, I shall try to find out more about it or why it is supposed to be necessary."

Enayat was born and grew up in Cairo, though her family is originally from upper Egypt, and she went to school for seven years. Both parents could read and write, and her father worked as a health assistant. She is the youngest of three sisters, all were circumcised before age 8. **Enayat had worked as a housekeeper for years, and when she was asked if she remembers when she was circumcised, she replied, "How can I forget!" This is the story Enayat told about her operation:**

"I knew about the event and my mother kept telling me once you are circumcised you will grow taller and prettier, it helps a girl develop. On the morning of the operation the daya who came to our home told me not to be afraid. Her assistant caught hold of me and twisted my arms under my legs in a brutal way and held me down. I screamed from fear and pain. At first I was unable to urinate and when I finally did it hurt and burned. Every morning and evening my mother took care of the wound.

I stayed in bed five days, and for seven days I was given chicken for lunch, my mother said it was good for me. Later I learned they had cut off all of the clitoris.

I was afraid what would happen at my wedding night. When the hymen was broken my blood stained the sheets and a towel: my mother and family saw the blood stains and were reassured. During the earlier years of my married life, my husband had intercourse with me almost every night. I thought it was wrong, I felt nothing, but had to submit out of duty. I came from a strict family; sex was never mentioned.

When I was about to circumcise my eldest daughter at the age of 8, an enlightened lady whom I met explained all the fallacies regarding the practice and advised me against it. I persuaded my husband, and my girls were spared. My neighbors followed my example.

I am convinced it is wrong, and I know of many cases of bleeding after the operation. One girl in our neighborhood bled to death, though she was taken to the hospital. The parents were taken to court and penalized. Unfortunately, the operation is now done in secret, and serious cases are not taken to the hospital for fear of punishment. I think it is wrong. I shall not have my daughters operated."

In all Egyptian hospitals one can find bleeding girls terribly injured and permanently damaged as a result of excision; but the parents and dayas are rarely prosecuted, and usually the whole affair is hushed up.

Halima is a 34-year-old mother of seven children, including three daughters. A Moslem from a traditional close-knit family in Cairo, she has never gone to school or learned to read, though television is now available throughout that populous city. **Halima supports all traditions, and is a strong advocate of excision:**

"Excision is important for all women, so there is no confusion between the sexes. Every woman to be a real woman must be excised. Believe me, a man gets much more pleasure from a woman who has no clitoris. I was excised when I was about 6 years old. I was the first daughter, and I was dressed up like a little bride. Yes, it did hurt, and I was put to bed and given all kinds of special foods. The clitoris which was cut off was rolled up with salt and put in a little bag and tied to my arm for a week like a bracelet. Everyone in the family took care of me; I was glad to be the center of attention.

My wedding night was also very special: my mother, my mother-in-law and my aunt were with me, and my husband deflowered me with a finger wrapped in a handkerchief. The bloody handkerchief was then shown to all the relatives waiting outside our bed chamber including all my brothers. We are a large family and everyone came to celebrate; they played music and tam tams. I now have three daughters and of course they all will be excised to make them into real women. The operation also helps them grow. No one wants girls who are like boys!

Of course, my husband is all for it because girls who are not excised are wild, they run around and are always excited. Everyone in our neighborhood has their daughters done, no one wants hypersexual girls. All our Egyptian girls must be excised because it is good for them; only the foreigners are not. "

Most of the girls subjected to FGM are never informed of what is going to be done to them and have no idea about the real consequences of the operations, let alone the dangers involved. When asked later about the operations, many talk about the terrible pain. But most women never really learn the truth about the psychological damage. To remove or literally cut out the nerve center that is one of the mainsprings of life, is not limited to the physical damage sustained: it also mutilates the spirit and zest for life and living, the carefree enjoyment by the young. Removing the feeling in the most sensitive genital area and nerve center of the female body, especially at an early age, impairs all ability to feel and respond to all sensory stimulation.

No one has ever examined the long-term psychological results because it is too difficult and the results may be too painful for all involved. What little research on the psychological effects that has been done mostly examined social factors rather than long-range psychological influences, and did not arrive at any conclusions.

However, the effect of the trauma of the operations and the social implications are known, including by fathers, as the reasons given for the operations show: these operations, it is claimed, are necessary to make the girls calm down and quiet so they are easy to manage and obedient. It is said that a girl who is not operated is wild, she cannot be controlled, she will disgrace her family, she cannot control her sexuality. **The operation is used to break the spirit of the girl child to make her into an obedient slave** of the man who pays the highest brideprice and therefore has the right to use and abuse her in any way he wants. The mutilations prepare her for a life of pain and abuse by the man selected by her father to use her body to produce children for him. Her consent is never even a question; **she has no will of her own, she is the wholly owned property of men.**

Women are led to believe the damaging myths they are told to persuade them to undergo the mutilations and/or to force these "important traditions" on their daughters. They are told these operations are "necessary" for a whole host of reasons that differ according to the ethnic group but continue to be proclaimed as truths despite all known biological facts. The reasons include: to have children; to satisfy the husband; to be a real woman; to be accepted by the community; to remove something ugly; to be clean and for a woman's health; to be beautiful; to increase fertility; to prevent the clitoris from harming the baby during birth or damaging the husband during intercourse, and much more. The many reasons given are an amazing example of traditional imagination which, unhampered by any scientific knowledge, engages in astounding conjectures. **But the tragic facts is that in the absence of biological facts or realistic information these myths are all believed.**

Egypt has the largest population program, which was started more than 15 years ago and is now fully supported by the Government: **it is funded by the US Agency for International Development (USAID).** But despite millions spent annually, the Egyptian population is growing relentlessly in a country that has huge deserts and very little arable land. Most of the population lives on imported food subsidized by the US. Yet despite intensive efforts to limit population growth which continue today, a large percentage of women still cannot read, which is the first door that needs to be opened to enable women to control their fertility - the most effective way to reduce population growth.

Television has also been enlisted in the population control efforts and is watched by most of the urbanized population. But despite the many well-financed media efforts **all programs have excluded any mention of FGM,** though, as documented above, a majority of girls continue to be mutilated, confirming that women are not in control of their lives.

A survey made at a low-income area family planning clinic in Cairo found that not only were most of the clients excised, but **the trained family planning women workers employed at this establishment were excised themselves, and had, or were planning to have, their own daughters excised! Evidently the dangers and damage to women's health due to FGM were never discussed during the training.** This appalling situation is financially supported by USAID, which pays for training programs. The population programs of USAID have refused to even acknowledge the existence of FGM in Egypt, though their contractors have implemented multimillion-dollar population programs in Egypt for years. USAID **ignores the health of women by failing to teach prevention of FGM,** as I have stated repeatedly in my Congressional testimonies. (See the chapter on Politics.)

KENYA

In 1982, while traveling around rural Kenya during the season when girls are excised, President Daniel arap Moi was told that seven young girls had died that past week in that area as the result of excision. It was then, while speaking at a large gathering, that he proclaimed that as long as he was president he would not allow little girls to die in that dreadful way. He followed up this speech with an official order to prohibit the practice.

This was a most important positive step and a radical beak with the past - especially since it was followed up with a prohibition to all hospitals to do the operations. But it has not stopped the practice as it was not followed by an education and information campaign. This was recently confirmed by a research report published by the largest women's organization of Kenya, **Maendeleo Ya Wanawake,** * which found that FGM is practiced in a large part of the country including in hospitals. (See chapter on Politics.)

The issue of FGM was already politicized in Kenya during colonial times when some missionary physicians strongly opposed the practice on health grounds. **President Kenyatta, Kenya's revered first leader who became president-for-life in 1962** and was the head of the Kikuyu, the leading tribe of Kenya, strongly supported the mutilation of all girls during his lifetime, **declaring that no Kikuyu would ever think of marrying a woman who was not excised.** His support of FGM had great influence all over Africa, deterring for years all efforts to protect millions of little girls from this terrible butchery.

Since the Kikuyu hold the political leadership in Kenya, FGM was excluded from all discussion by the women leaders, including one of the most influential ones, **Eddah Gachukia, M.P. Her appointment to Parliament, the basis of much of her power, was made by Kenyatta.** As head of the National Council of Women of Kenya and leader of the Kenyan delegation at the 1980 UN Mid-Decade Conference in Copenhagen, Gachukia and most Kenyan women leaders claimed that the mutilations were being abandoned. At a meeting at the Copenhagen Forum, the Kenyan women leaders stated that the facts were not known and therefore they could not talk about it; **but they had blocked, and continued to block, all efforts to do the necessary research to establish the facts.**

Excision was never seriously discussed in Kenya, while every year scores of little girls died as a result of the mutilations, as reported by Kenyan papers, and many thousands were operated on, often in drastic ways, including infibulation. At the UN Mid-Decade **Conference Forum in Nairobi, in 1985, when FGM was discussed by the Inter-African Committee** in a series of overflow meetings, **the Kenyan women leaders never came** or said a word, and many of them are silent even now. Therefore the program that was finally started three years ago by **Maendeleo Ya Wanawake,** * which reaches women in rural areas, represents real change.

In 1992, at the end of the first two phases of research, conducted with technical help from Appropriate Technology in Health (PATH) and financed by Population Action International (PAI) as well as the Ford Foundation, a **"Dissemination Workshop"** was held in Nairobi to make the findings known among a large number of groups and institutions concerned with women's development and health. **The research findings showed that in the four districts where investigations were conducted, 90 percent of the women were mutilated. It was also documented that FGM is practiced in the hospitals.**

Recommendations for actions in the three major areas of health care, communication and policy/law were discussed. Resolutions were adopted to pursue eradication by integrating efforts in many areas, adopting a multi-pronged approach including contacting various relevant ministries. Phase III of the program, to implement strategies based on the findings to create awareness about the harmful effects of FGM, has recently begun in the four districts where the research was done. But as everyone at the Dissemination Workshop agreed, **it will take time to change ingrained ideas and convictions** - especially since even in Kenya, which is far ahead of most other African countries, literacy is still quite low in rural areas, especially among women.

---

*Maendeleo Ya Wanawake Women's Organization (MYWO) - "Women's Progress," P.O. Box 44412, Nairobi, Kenya; Leah W. Muuya, program manager. "Report on a Dissemination Workshop on Female Circumcision." See **WIN NEWS**, Vol. 20, No. 3, Summer 1994, pp. 127-29, and **The HOSKEN REPORT** chapter on "Women and Health."

Over the years, many in Kenya have spoken on FGM, including the press, even though the prestigious National Council of Women chose to ignore the ongoing mutilations.

Midwives in Kenya, as elsewhere in Africa, are most knowledgeable on what is going on regarding FGM, especially in the rural areas. Kenya has a much better health system, begun by the British in colonial times, than francophone West Africa where I also visited hospital maternities. At present, AIDS is spreading rapidly all over Kenya, though facts are hard to obtain as the Government is concerned that such information might damage the tourist trade on which Kenya depends. It is clear that FGM contributes to the spread of AIDS, even though this is rarely discussed. **In addition, polygamy, promiscuity by men and widespread rape*** especially of the young, as reported almost daily by the press, result in the spread of AIDS and all sexually transmitted diseases.

As elsewhere in Africa, men go to the towns, claiming they are looking for work, leaving women and children behind to do the hard labor of farming by themselves. Though most men don't find jobs in the towns they do get infected with AIDS, which they then bring to the rural areas when visiting their families. **A midwife describes traditional conditions in rural areas, which have changed little, as the investigations of Maendeleo also confirm:**

> "Circumcision is going on in the rural areas, especially among those who are still strong believers of our traditions and customs, such as the Kuria, Kisii, Masai, Suk, Nandi, Kipsigis and Kamba. The reason for circumcising is that the sexual urge will decrease, since the sensitive organ is cut off. Therefore she will not have sexual relations with a man before marriage. When married the excised woman will not have extramarital sexual relationships - thus keeping moral behavior in the society.
>
> Through my experience as midwife I have seen some mothers, especially those having children for the first time, having complications such as delay in second stage labor because of the excision scar the perineum cannot stretch to give room for the baby's head. . . An episiotomy has to be performed each time the woman gives birth; if not, there is a serious tear and this may involve also the rectum . . . sometimes these women end up with a fistula which causes incontinence and is very hard to repair. . . Also, the babies born of these women, especially if premature, often die of brain damage. Some babies are born dead because of delay in second stage if born at home without a qualified midwife. . . Bleeding is profuse in case of tears; the scars always form haematoma when bruised which is very painful . . ."

In the Kenyatta Hospital in Nairobi - the largest and best-equipped hospital in Kenya - **there is a constant waiting list of hundreds of women waiting to have a fistula repaired,** as this tear, which results in incontinence, makes them outcasts from their families.

A recent survey made at a girls' high school in the Tharaka region, east of Mount Kenya, showed that all the 16- to 21-year-old girls had already been mutilated. What is more, 78 out of the 97 surveyed stated that their future daughters also will be operated - but when asked about their granddaughters, 93 said no. Another investigation in the schools found a marked decrease in the number of mutilations close to Nairobi and other urban centers, as well as where strong campaigns against the practice had taken place in the past. **But in Roman Catholic schools, reflecting the conservative stand of that church, most of the girls were mutilated. An educator at a girls' school states:**

> "Unfortunately, little is being done in the area of sex education . . . Many schools were originally founded by missionaries and 'sex' just was not discussed in the classroom - it is a question of embarrassment, due to social/religious influences."

As a result of this embarrassment the younger generation is kept in ignorance, which for girls and women may often be fatal. Surveys made by population programs on young people's knowledge of human reproduction in **Nairobi teacher training colleges reported general confusion among their students about such matters.**

---

*In July 1991, the murder of 19 and rape of 71 teenage schoolgirls by their male classmates at a Catholic boarding school in Meru was reported around the world. The principal stated to the press: "The boys never meant any harm against the girls; they just wanted to rape." (See **WIN NEWS** Vol. 17, No. 4, Autumn 1991, pp. 37-39.)

A few years ago I offered the Minister of Primary Education of Kenya free copies of our **Childbirth Picture Books**, which explain reproduction in quite basic terms in pictures and are easy to understand by anyone. This offer was turned down under the pretext that the schools had no trained personnel to introduce these books. But, as I explained, no experts or trained professionals are needed to distribute these books - as our experience all over the world shows. **Most anyone, young or old, can figure out what the pictures mean and the text is easy to read, even by those with limited reading skills.***

The economic or financial implications of the mutilations as well as the brideprice act as incentives to continue these practices - which so greatly damage women. A women's publication in Nairobi states:

> "Brideprice operating in a money economy has come to acquire the qualities of a sale - it is now, more than ever before, the **price** of a woman. Greed and gain have led some parents to force their daughters to leave school, even if they are still very young, to wed rich elderly men for a fat brideprice . . . It is always argued by protagonists of brideprice that it protects the virtue of girls, and ensures stability of the marriage . . . But brideprice in reality is an anachronistic archaic custom that reduces women to merchandise and in an overtly polygamous society like Kenya it promotes inequality. . ."

Excision and/or infibulation traditionally are required by a husband-to-be who will not pay brideprice to the father otherwise. Hence fathers see to it that daughters are operated. But the operations cost money - indeed performing the mutilations is a lucrative business. The earnings of a circumcisor in Kenya can be considerable, so the midwives report:

> "The job usually is a family matter, young people learn the trade from their grandmothers and mothers. Circumcisors consider themselves to provide an important and respected service. The money is paid by the father of the girl in appreciation for services rendered . . ."

There are no other jobs in rural areas that pay a comparable income, though it is a seasonal occupation. But even here, the price paid to the circumcisor of boys, so the midwives report, is considerably higher than what is paid to women to cut girls.

The investigation by the Maendeleo women's organization produced some ambivalent and even contradictory opinions on circumcision expressed by different people - mothers, fathers, girls, boys and opinion leaders - in four separate rural communities and ethnic groups that practice FGM. Here are some of the ideas expressed:

> **"Mothers** who want to continue the practice claim that circumcised daughters had increased chances of getting married; parents of circumcised girls are honored and respected by their community; circumcised girls make obedient wives. Mothers who wanted the practice to continue lacked information about the hazards; a few mothers who knew the dangers wanted the operations to stop and felt that the practice was outdated, meaningless and dehumanizing . . .

> **Many of the girls** stated that the practice was good and should continue - they looked forward to it as a time of feasting, dancing, special treatment, presents. Marriage often follows the operation which means more celebrations. Some feared they would be ostracized by the community if not circumcised and would have childbirth problems. Others considered it dreadful, humiliating and dangerous; Many also know uncircumcised women who are married, educated and highly respected. . .

> **Many fathers** claimed that women wanted circumcision to continue, while they were opposed; others claimed uncircumcised women were unclean, rude and bossy . ."

Maendeleo at present is continuing to work on the development of their programs.

---

* **Women's International Network** publishes the **Childbirth Picture Books** in a number of languages with separate **Additions to Prevent Excision and Infibulation**. These books are also used in Kenya by several programs and groups with very good results. But they have never been introduced on a mass scale with "before" and "after" tests, to record the positive results, especially for school systems. Anyone interested in such a program and test should contact **WIN NEWS**.

ETHIOPIA

Aisha and her husband temporarily live in the US, but they expect to return to Ethiopia when political conditions are settled. She managed to escape from the war, because she was one of the very few women to get a good education. This is her story:

"My name is Aisha, my family lives in Ethiopia in a town in the eastern part of the country inhabited by people of Somali origin. When I started to go to school the girls talked about the presents they hoped to receive when they would undergo some mysterious operation. I did not know what they were talking about, so one day I asked my mother, but she was reluctant to answer and said I was too thin; she was afraid that there might be problems. But some months later she called the local midwife and invited the whole family and friends for the initiation of me and my little sister, age 5. **My mother told me to be brave, it will hurt, but every girl has to have it done to become a woman.** She prepared the whole house for the occasion and got beautiful clothes of satin with ribbons ready for us; there was perfume and incense and many sweets for the guests including my school friends.

The midwife and her helpers came before the guests; I was put on a table in a back room with my hands behind me, one woman opened my legs, two women held my left and right shoulders. I was determined to be courageous and happy because I knew something very special was about to happen, so the girls in school had said, though I did not know what. I had put a roll of cloth in my mouth so my friends who now were arriving in the yard would not hear me cry.

The midwife excisor, an old woman, took a little knife she had brought out of a special pocket and began the cutting. A piercing pain shook my whole thin body; the overwhelming pain of the cutting went on and on but I could not move as I was held down by strong hands. Finally the midwife began to sew me up. At last she closed my legs and tied them together with wide bandages after inserting a little stick so I would be able to urinate after the scar formed. I heard the noise of the celebration going on in the yard but I hurt too much and did not want to see anyone.

I had to lie still for what seemed an endless time. Finally, many days later I was allowed to stand up and hop about like a bird with my legs closed, holding onto a large stick. All that time I only ate some rice and drank as little as possible as urination caused dreadful pains. Then one day I stumbled and fell and the scar broke. My mother forced me to have it resewn though I was afraid of the pain. But she said I could never get married if I was not closed and all girls must have it done. **Not until I went to university in Europe, years later, did I find out that girls in most countries of the world are not closed and never go through these terrible operations.**

When you start menstruating more problems may come. Fortunately I did not have much trouble though I had great pain each month. But my younger sister had blood clots because the blood could not come out and hardened and caused constant pain. With some girls it gets so bad that they have to go to the midwife to be opened and have the blood clots taken out.

The next problems arise when you get married. **According to tradition, the husband is supposed to open the bride using his penis as a battering ram.** The bride is chosen by his family and is inspected to make sure she is properly closed. But first the bride price must be paid in full. Fortunately this did not happen to me personally as I was sent abroad to study, and before I got married to a fellow student I went to a surgeon who opened me under anesthesia. **But usually it is an old woman from the husband's family who cuts open the bride with a knife - recently a razor blade - and then the new husband has to have intercourse frequently through the bleeding wound to keep it from closing again.**

I assisted at the marriage of a very good friend of mine when I came home, a beautiful woman. She was never even asked when she was married to a stranger her father had picked. She was made to produce children without being asked; she was used like an object and became like a vegetable and never revolted. She was literally dead - an ideal wife from the prevailing male view in our society. I have a little feeling left, but I don't like sex; **I wonder what it is like to really feel like my friends at the university who tried to tell me about what I have lost forever.**"

NIGERIA

In Nigeria, the most populous English-speaking country in Africa, the issue of FGM has been discussed for years and often quite publicly, including in the press. In the late 1970's, Esther Ogunmodede published an article in **The Drum,** a national magazine: **"How much longer will we allow our girls to be brutalized in this barbaric way?"** The article stirred up a large response; letters by readers debating excision - pro and con - continued to be published for two years in a huge letter-writing campaign in which many people did not hesitate to contribute their opinions.

After giving the background facts and explaining the operations and their health effects, **Ogunmodede cites two women who were operated on as children. Jumai, the first one, has this to say:**

> "Early one morning when I woke up, I wondered what all that boiling water was for. Nobody said anything, but by 6 a.m. our local barber had arrived; the elders in our house gathered. I was getting scared as I was only 10 years old. My elderly aunt undressed me and blindfolded me with a scarf. I was then forcibly held down and my legs pulled apart while the barber/surgeon did his work. I was screaming until I could scream no more, and passed out. When I came around, I could not urinate for hours. It was sheer hell when I did."

Ogunmodede then explains that among the Hausa in the Moslem north of Nigeria, local barbers do all surgery, including tribal marks and excision.

In the other story, Risikat, a young law student, relates what happened to her, after asserting that under no circumstances will any of her daughters be operated on:

> "It took five people to hold me down, and I was only 8. All the neighbors had gathered and were shouting advice to the olola and jeering at me for lacking courage. In the struggle, the olola cut the wrong section, which has left me permanently damaged. It was a nightmare that still remains with me today."

The "olola" families are the traditional circumcisers among the Yoruba, an ethnic group of many millions of people who live in the southern and western part of Nigeria. **Excision is an inherited trade in Nigeria and much of Africa, which is passed on from mother to daughter; for circumcision of boys from father to son.** In a few areas, men do some of the surgery on girls as well, especially in towns. Barbers do the operations not only in Nigeria but also in Egypt. Ogunmodede tried to find out why these operations continue to be performed even today:

> "No one to whom I spoke could tell me why, though the easiest and commonest answer is that it is our 'custom and tradition,' the shield behind which we hide the more hideous and inexplicable of our practices. . .
>
> Most children become so uncontrollable with bewilderment and panic that 'accidents' occur, resulting in terrible injuries. Why then do we subject our own daughters to the same horrors?"

The letters sent by readers following the article's publication give an unusually frank view of a cross-section of Nigerians. Both women and men state their opinions about FGM quite publicly and without hesitation :

Mr. D.I., Calabar, "How Esther Got it Wrong":

"The ultimate aim of a girl is to grow up and become useful to her husband and the society to which she belongs. Taking a closer look at women in the United States, for example, women there are very impetuous. In their desperate drive for sexual satisfaction they cause irreparable harm to their husbands. Even in Nigeria, the few uncircumcised women tend to be brutal and wicked in dealing with their husbands."

Ms. O.B., School of Nursing, Ife, "End This Barbarism":

"Our forefathers practiced what I term 'facial decoration' with tribal marks as part of their cultural components. How many of you advocates of female circumcision for reasons of 'culture' would want to mark the faces of your children? I agree with Esther Ogunmodede: the act is brutal and barbaric. It should be stopped."

Mr. A.J.A., circumciser:

"Circumcision is the profession of my family. I have built two houses with the proceeds from circumcision and I have several children in different schools. I circumcise both males and females, and inscribe tribal marks on people who want them. I have dealt with almost all ethnic groups in Nigeria.

On the question of circumcision for female children: Our forefathers believed in it, and there must always be tradition. What damage does it do to the female organ? As far as I am concerned, it does no harm. Even the Quran supports circumcision."

Mr. J.A., "An Unhealthy Archaic Tradition":

"Reading the opinions of fellow Nigerians on this matter, one is bound to conclude that most of us either do not know or do not understand the evil effects of female circumcision. Apart from the pain that women suffer from the crude knives of the so-called native circumcisers, they are subjected to nothing but agony whenever they dare get close to their loved ones. This itself leads to frustrated sexual as well as married lives.

It is beyond my comprehension how a man or a woman could postulate that a woman has no right to enjoy sex, if that is what they mean by women being 'too sexy,' and that her clitoris should be removed. To male chauvinists who argue that only men have the right to enjoy sex, I say what is sauce for the gander is sauce for the goose.

Let us ask ourselves how much men would like it if the case were reversed, if men were castrated by the native 'circumcisors' so that they would not be 'too sexy' and run after women?. . . It is high time the African women claimed their rights as human beings, not as second-class citizens. . ."

Mr. M.A., businessman:

"In the Yoruba tribe, circumcision is just like tribal marks. It is part of custom and tradition left for us by our fathers. I have heard that some tribes in Nigeria don't circumcise their girls, but in my own tribe in Kwara State we do circumcise our girls. Naturally, uncircumcised girls are more sexy and if they are in such a state they may lose interest in more important things like their education. . ."

Ms. T.M., Miss Nigeria:

"Biologically, the clitoris is the most sensitive organ of a woman, and that was why parents of past days made sure they cut it off - to stop their girls from being wayward. It is cruel and it should not be encouraged. As for me, I will never have it done to my daughters."

Dr. Bertha Johnson, a psychiatrist who lives in Lagos and participated in the World Health Organization seminar in 1979 in Khartoum as the head of the Nigerian delegation, explains the basic attitudes and motivations of her society:

"As a psychiatrist, I am aware that people here in Nigeria have an obsession about children. Infertility is a terrible problem for women who become very depressed if they cannot have children. If you are infertile, you are useless as the only purpose of an African woman's life is to have as many children as possible. For men also, to have a child is essential as his manhood is involved. . .

Among the Yoruba who live in this part of the country (Lagos), it is believed that excision is necessary to dampen the sexuality of women, and to prevent stillbirths because if the clitoris touches the head of the child during birth, the child will die. Hence it is removed before marriage.

There is still a double standard in our society. The families of the husband and the wife interfere as according to tradition they should settle quarrels between couples; but this often creates worse problems. There is a lot of wife beating, yet an abused wife gets no help from her family. If a man would try to beat me he would not do it twice. If more women would feel that way, wife beating would disappear in Africa."

The health problems of women as well as the many dangerous and damaging traditional practices that continue today all over Nigeria, resulting in some of the highest maternal mortality anywhere, are discussed in the book **Women's Health Issues in Nigeria,** * written and published by Nigerian women professionals. The book provides a stunning insight into many of the problems that affect women in this large and diverse society. Mere Nakateregga Kisekka, the editor, states in the introduction:

> "Women die more from pregnancy and childbirth-related problems than from any other cause. . . Data show that 80% of complications resulting in maternal deaths are associated with haemorrhage. . . Obstructed labour features as the antecedent event in the major causes of maternal mortality. . .

> Women are subject to and inculcated into oppressive traditional values. . .Women's low socioeconomic status renders them powerless in decision-making even on matters as vital and personal as their health, sexuality, and fertility. The majority of dangerous traditional practices affect women's reproductive health."

Many of these dangerous traditions - most of them related to childbearing - are discussed and documented by different researchers that contributed to the book. Despite the importance given by men to fathering children, the male decision makers, due to neglect of health education and the failure to provide the most essential hospital and childbirth services, **have made childbearing into the most dangerous occupation of women.**

There is no excuse. Nigeria can afford decent maternity clinics and services, but as again documented in this book, **since all decisions are made by men no money is spent on the urgent health needs of women, especially maternity services and health education** to stop some of the devastating traditional practices.

The Inter-African Committee of Nigeria, headed by Dr. Irene Thomas, the first female physician of Nigeria, has undertaken the enormous job of organizing an information campaign to stop FGM and to train traditional birth attendants and teach women to go out into their communities to campaign against the many harmful and dangerous traditional practices. **Ms. E.M. Alabi, the coordinator of the IAC of Nigeria,** a midwife with extensive training and field experience, has organized training programs and has campaigned all over the country. The remarkable, relentless work of the IAC is reported in their health magazine, **Your Task.** **

Aside from genital mutilation, which is still practiced by more than half of the Nigerian population - more than 50 million people - in that rapidly growing country, many other damaging practices prevail including "gishiri cuts" - cuts into the vagina of young girls. There also are a whole list of food tabus especially for pregnant women which eliminate the most nutritional foods a woman needs in order to have a healthy baby and sustain a pregnancy. **The list of dangerous superstitions and damaging practices related to childbirth goes on and on, as researched by Alabi, who teaches all over Nigeria** to change such damaging customs. More about this is documented in **WIN NEWS** and in the chapters on Nigeria and "Women and Health" of **The HOSKEN REPORT.**

The real problem is that the Nigerian Government, and the men who make the decisions, have utterly neglected health care for the rapidly growing population, as is documented in the above-cited book on women's health and by **Ms. Alabi, who states:**

> "Nigeria, which has a large population . . . is faced with serious limitations such as inadequate health facilities and trained personnel. As a result, 70 percent of childbearing women depend on traditional birth attendants, traditional healers and herbalists for their health care, who are usually illiterates without any formal training in delivery procedures and with strong beliefs in supernatural powers. . ."

* **Women's Health Issues in Nigeria**, edited by Dr. Mere Nakateregga Kisekka, Coordinator, Center for Social and Economic Research, Ahmadu Bello University, Zaria/ Kaduna State, Nigeria. (See **WIN NEWS**, Vol. 19, No. 3, Summer 1993, pp. 37/38.)

** **Your Task - Health Magazine of the Inter-African Committee (IAC) of Nigeria on Harmful Traditional Practices**, P.O. Box 6051, Lagos, Nigeria; Dr. Irene Thomas, president.

SENEGAL

In Senegal, which is located at the westernmost tip of Africa, the leading ethnic group, the Wolofs, do not practice FGM. This is exactly the opposite of Kenya, where the political leaders are the Kikuyu, and their former leader, President-for-Life Kenyatta, was the most vocal advocate for FGM in Kenya and all over Africa. The question is: does Senegal therefore offer more protection against FGM for women?

This is hard to answer. Since FGM does not concern the leadership and their families directly, it has never been a political issue as in Kenya; for the most part it has been entirely ignored. Indeed, until quite recently, the facts on where FGM is practiced or by whom had never been researched or established until a comprehensive study on **Excision in Senegal** was made by Marie Helene Mottin-Sylla and published by ENDA* in Dakar in 1990.

Due to urbanization and especially immigration to Dakar from all rural areas, it was known to the midwives working in the maternity hospitals in Dakar who practices what type of mutilation. **Maternities in Dakar, as in other capitals in Africa, not only get all the complicated deliveries but women from all ethnic groups deliver there. By going to maternities all over Africa, I was able to establish these facts long before any detailed research studies were made.**

Dakar was the seat of the French Government-in-exile during World War II which has left a permanent imprint on this city. In colonial times Dakar was the French administrative center for West Africa. **In no other city of Africa is the contrast between modern life and African tradition more glaring than in Dakar.** Therefore, Dakar has long been a magnet for enterprising Africans from all over West Africa.

While women in Dakar seem very sophisticated and have some access to jobs and a few opportunities to gain a little political power, in the rural areas nothing has changed and traditional life goes on much as in the past. **Illiteracy is especially high among women in Senegal, but very little is being done by the Government to change this situation.** As elsewhere in Africa, women do much of the agricultural work and are overburdened with heavy daily chores. FGM is still practiced in many rural areas, and polygamy is widespread among the very traditional 94 percent Moslem population.

Perhaps this dichotomy explains how a woman who held a well-paid media job in Dakar turned out to be one of the most vocal proponents of FGM at the 1980 Mid-Decade Conference for Women in Copenhagen. **Marie Angelique Savane, by praising FGM as an essential African tradition, attracted great press attention to herself and was published all over Europe and the US by those eagerly speaking for culture and tradition.** "What are we going to put in place of initiation that every girl looks forward to?" she asked, accusing all those working to stop it, including me, of "cultural imperialism." Savane collected her rewards by gaining enormous media coverage and, finally, a much coveted administrative job at the UN in Geneva where male African officials have much influence.

The recent claim made by a Sudanese expatriate living in the US, Nahid Toubia, is in the same category. **She stated that FGM is chosen by women to make themselves more desirable to men and compared it to breast implants.** Toubia made this offensive statement on women very publicly on national television in the US, in a discussion on FGM with UNICEF director James Grant, which attracted a great deal of attention.

In some rural areas of southeastern Senegal FGM is practiced in quite extreme ways, including infibulation. As Mottin-Sylla discovered when organizing some meetings, presumably to introduce new ideas in the very traditional rural areas, **the influential rural Moslem leaders firmly insisted that FGM was a religious command and required by the Koran as an absolute obligation,** and they categorically opposed all change. Of course, no women were allowed to speak. Providing traditionalists an opportunity to voice their ideas publicly is not the road to change - on the contrary.

Overall, about 20 percent of the Senegalese population subject their daughters to FGM, according to Mottin-Sylla's research. Since the vast majority of the Senegalese are Moslem it is obviously not a religious practice but an ethnic one.

***Excision au Senegal**, Marie Helene Mottin-Sylla, ENDA, B.P. 3370, Dakar, Senegal.

A "Case History on Senegal" is included in **The HOSKEN REPORT** which provides extensive documentation of what is very briefly summarized here.

The coast around Dakar is replete with luxury hotels where French and European women bathe topless on the beaches of the winter resorts. None of them know about the plight of the little African girls who have the misfortune to be born into ethnic groups that claim all girls must be brutally mutilated or they are not acceptable to a husband. Despite being closer to France than any other West African country and despite years of development programs of all kinds, the vast majority of women of Senegal continue to be illiterate.

Most rural women are overburdened with heavy household work starting in childhood; as girls they have no chance to learn or get any education that could open access to another life; they are often still isolated in their fathers' and husbands' houses with no chance to make contact with the outside world. It is that terrible prison constructed by men to hold onto their "property" that is the cause and reason why development will never succeed until and unless women are freed from their manmade bonds. **Little or nothing is done to improve education for girls, which was already completely neglected in colonial times by the French.** Despite the superficial French-inspired sophistication displayed in Dakar, Senegal is desperately poor. The official literacy rate is 28 percent, which means that more than 80 percent women cannot read.

Some of the women's stories below, as told to Mottin-Sylla, shed some light on the attitudes of a society where these practices continue to persist even though they are neither promoted by the majority nor by the political leadership as they used to be in Kenya. **Perhaps one reason is the terribly damaging isolation of women,** and this applies not only to Africa but to much of the developing world.

M. M., a Serere who is 25 years old, explains the customs of her ethnic group:

"With us, excision is directly connected with initiation and tradition in an Islamized environment. The girls stay with the excisor for three days. On the fourth day the operation is done early in the morning with scissors while two women helpers hold each girl - one the head and shoulders, the other the legs. Afterward the girls are divided up into those who have cried and those who were courageous - one group gets white armbands, the other red ones, and the excisor gets a chicken. To stop the bleeding and make the wound heal a concoction of leaves is boiled and put on the wound as well as nut butter, and the girls have to sit in hot water."

A young woman student in Dakar relates what happened to her:

"The reason for the operation typically is religious. I was 9 years old when it was done to me. I remember everything. I was taken to the excisor and told she was my aunt. After entering the house I was amazed when some women held me down and opened my legs. I got really frightened when the aunt took out a knife which she first put in boiling water and then she cut my clitoris off. I felt a terrible pain all over and thought I was dying. The excisor put some paste that burned between my legs. I was told I must push my legs together as hard as I could and not to move.

I was terrified, and I think this practice was invented to dehumanize women. The very thought of it still makes me ill. Under no circumstances will I ever have my daughter excised because it is a permanent handicap for personal development."

At the Bambara, girls are excised at an early age:

"We are Moslems and that is why we practice excision. It is done at a very young age, much as with the Peuls. Most of the time the tip of the clitoris is cut off; the aunt of the child selects a competent excisor. On the appointed day the girl is taken to the grandparents for their blessing, then she is excised together with other girls of the same age. During the operation loud incantations are chanted. Only after the wound is healed the aunt takes the girl back from the excisor's house and gives her new clothes. Due to this 'purification' once the girl reaches puberty she will be greatly respected. The excisor is paid with locally made soap."

A 30-year-old Wolof dressmaker explains what was done to her:

"In our society it is necessary to conform to tradition. I was excised the day before I was married. Just when I was going to be taken to my husband, the old women from the neighborhood who helped me to get ready for the wedding discovered that I was not excised as Wolofs do not practice this. They called an expert on this matter, and she told me that if I wanted my marriage to last and have children, it was absolutely necessary to do it. Then the women grabbed me and held me tight while they cut off my clitoris. I bled terribly, and fainted. The women to stop the bleeding put some compresses on the area of some sticky stuff, they also gave me something to put into my vagina. Sexual relations have been very painful for me, therefore, I try to avoid them. I had a very difficult delivery."

Infibulation is practiced by the Toucouleur, as a woman who was operated explains:

"Because virginity is considered sacred, infibulation is added to excision. That is, the flesh on each side of the big lips is held together and fused to form a scar over the entrance of the vagina. When I was excised they also closed the entrance to my vagina because my fiance was away on a trip. I was taken to the excisor who told me I have to open my legs in order to become a woman. And I must not cry too much to gain the respect of my fiance. I was held by two women so I could not move. The excisor wound a string around my clitoris and tightened it; then she cut off everything. I was overwhelmed by the burning pain. Then she took a needle and string and sewed the bleeding small lips together. I was so exhausted from this ordeal I could not move when they told me to get up. After two weeks she took out the string and all that remained was a scar formed by the dried blood."

A young Halpulaar woman who has gone to school speaks about excision:

"In Halpulaar, excision means purification - because if a child grows up without being excised, she is not only impure but she is the offspring of a polluted mother. She is rejected by the whole community and the very idea that a girl should not be excised is blasphemous! In order to make a girl faithful when she later gets married, it is necessary to amputate a part of herself. A girl who is not excised means that she is not respected and this will make her a second-class person. She has to be respectful of her parents and her future parents-in-law. She becomes a member of the adult community only after she is excised and assumes her place in society. The excisor, after the operation, uses all kinds of incantations to chase away the evil spirits; goat dung and nut butter are used on the wound for healing purposes. One has to pay the excisor eight pounds of rice and some soap."

Excision at the Soninke is required to become accepted in the community

"In the region of Fatick girls about 7 or 8 go to stay with the excisor. The day of the excision a big hole is dug in the ground, the girl takes off all her clothes and sits down in the hole with her back against the slope. Two women take hold of her arms and legs after bringing scissors, hot water and herbs that we prepared the night before. The excisor recites some incantations to ward off evil spirits, then cuts off the clitoris with the scissors and waits till the blood has stopped running into the sandy hole. Then she wipes the girl with hot water. A few hours later she puts the herbs on the wound. The excisor gets 200 francs and some soap."

At sunrise each morning in Dakar, the call of the muezzin is broadcast over the city from the mosques. Dakar has the appearance of a modern Western city, with handsome tree-planted avenues lined with cafes, and seems a very unlikely place for the practice of such damaging mutilations of children. Yet mutilations take place in many quarters of the city and nothing at all is said or done.

Women are not important in Senegal or other African societies; they are regarded as property of men. It is strange that the very African men who most loudly complain about racism, discrimination and colonialism, are utterly blind to the fact that they themselves practice the most damaging discrimination, sexism, abuse and violence against their own mothers, wives, daughters and sisters. **Worst of all, they do not even comprehend that what they do is utterly destructive to their own society.**

MALI

This description of initiation is by a young woman from Mali. She left her village to get an education which enables her to take a critical look at her experience and society:

"I remember every detail of this terrible affair. In our village it is the custom that several girls of the same age, about 9 to 12 years old, are operated on at the same time. This takes place at the house of an excisor. The village people come together to celebrate this occasion. The night before the drums were beaten until late.

Very early in the morning, two of my favorite aunts took me to the house of the excisor, an old woman from the blacksmith caste. In Mali, the women from this caste traditionally do genital operations, both clitoridectomy and infibulation.

Once inside the house of the operator I became terribly frightened, though I had been assured that it would not hurt. I did not know what excision meant though I had seen some girls who had been excised walking along, their backs were bent and they scarcely could hold themselves up. I was told to lie down on a mat on the floor. Immediately, some big hands fastened themselves on my thin legs and opened them wide. I raised my head, but two women held me down to the floor, I could not move.

I felt something being sprinkled on my genital area. Later, I learned this was sand, which is supposed to make excision easier. I tried to escape but they held me tight. I was terrified. Suddenly, some fingers pulled on my genital organs. A searing pain pierced me through and through. The excisor cut and cut: it took an interminable time, I felt as if I were being torn to pieces. The rule says that one must not cry during this operation. But I screamed and cried, and I was bleeding all over. Finally the operator put a mixture of herbs and butter on the wound to arrest the bleeding - I have never felt any pain as overwhelming as this. . .

Next the women who had held me down let go of me; but I couldn't get up. The voice of the operator called: 'It is finished. You can get up. You see, it didn't hurt much.' With the help of two women, I was put on my feet. I was made to walk to where the other girls who had been excised before me were waiting. Under the orders of the women in charge we were pushed to join a group of villagers who had gathered for this occasion to see us dance. I can't tell you how I felt.

I was burning all over. In tears, I tried to hop about a little, together with the other girls. We all were bleeding and hysterical from pain while being forced to dance. I shall always remember the terror of this monstrous affair, my friends and I with blood running down our legs and writhing in pain, being forced to jump around in a cloud of dust surrounded by gleeful clapping villagers. Then everything began to reel about me. I remember nothing more.

When I came to, I was stretched out in a hut with several people around me. Later, the most terrible moments of my life were when I had to urinate. It took a whole month before I healed. When I was well again, I was ridiculed by all the villagers because they said I wasn't courageous."

The official literacy rate in Mali for men and women is 10 percent, according to the latest statistics. **Since far fewer women than men learn to read, about 95 percent of women are illiterate** in this country, which is 90 percent Moslem.

Mali is one of the poorest landlocked countries in the world, where structural adjustment policies imposed by the WB/IMF (World Bank/International Monetary Fund) have further increased poverty and have made a terrible impact, especially on the lives of women. Both education and health care have been drastically cut back in an effort by the present government to pay for debts incurred by previous ones - mostly dictatorships. **As elsewhere, women are the principal victims of the cutbacks though they have been excluded from governmental decisions responsible for those debts.**

The WB/IMF austerity measures are dramatically expressed in the lack of health services, for instance, at the maternity of the Gabriel Toure Hospital, the largest city hospital of Bamako. At successive visits over the years to the maternity of this hospital, I could observe the cutbacks in services and equipment for myself.

The few midwives left at the Gabriel Toure Hospital told me they had nothing to work with, not even rubber gloves or scissors let alone any drugs, and their salaries had not been paid for months. Most maternity staff had left, the huge dark-tiled halls of the hospital were almost empty, and the stone stairs - all built in colonial times - had not been washed for a long time. **"We have no soap," the midwives said, "let alone anything else we need."** A surgeon I met in the yard told me that "I was just starting an operation when the electricity supply failed and the lights went off."

The Gabriel Toure Hospital maternity is the largest one in Mali and the only one that could take care of complicated deliveries that often result from genital mutilation. No wonder the maternal mortality rate is increasing. **But all the internationally-sponsored Safe Motherhood programs by WHO, the World Bank and USAID totally ignore the very existence of genital mutilation - the cause of thousands of unnecessary deaths in childbirth.** Yet these programs waste millions annually on high-level conferences held in luxury hotels all over the world, including in Africa. (See **The HOSKEN REPORT** chapter on "The Politics of FGM - A Conspiracy of Silence.")

In Mali, though infibulation is not usually done by using fastening devices as in Sudan or Somalia, the drastic operations often have the same result of closing the entrance to the vagina by tying the legs of the mutilated girls and keeping them immobilized until the wound has healed. Thus scar tissue accomplishes the same results of infibulation, which makes unassisted childbirth impossible. Often women are in labor for days, unable to break the hardened scars after having been impregnated through a tiny opening. **I talked to the midwives at the Gabriel Toure maternity:**

> "Many women have their vaginas closed, and this creates great problems in delivery. Unless there is skilled help to cut the obstruction, both mother and baby die. But no one attributes such a death to its real cause. Most often, it is said that an evil spirit is responsible for any problems in childbirth, or even the mother herself. She must have done something wrong, and so she is being punished.

> Some of the women who come to the maternity are very young. Some are married even before they menstruate. The other day a girl came to deliver; she was barely 14. We discovered it was her third child. Polygamy is widely practiced, and the younger wives are integrated into the labor force of the village household as soon as the brideprice is arranged and they have recovered from the excision. Their work is needed by the older wives, and they learn to take care of the children before they have any themselves."

Excision in Mali is traditionally a coming-of-age rite; a girl is not accepted into adult society until she is excised nor can she get married. **And marriage in Mali, much as in the rest of Africa, is an absolute requirement; there is no alternative, nor to childbearing.** Yet everywhere in Africa, though men are obsessed with having more and more children, who are regarded as status symbols and a boost of manhood, the maternity hospitals and services are totally neglected.

Men claim childbirth is a women's affair, and if women die in the process the men don't care - they can always purchase another wife. Making more children is no problem for men. **Thus all the male-dominated governments of Africa have neglected all maternity and health services for women which rank lowest on their national agenda and budget,** leading to a huge maternal mortality especially where such practices as excision and infibulation still continue.

There are many other traditions that terribly damage women's health, but it continues to be claimed, especially by international development programs of United Nations agencies and USAID, that "cultural traditions must be preserved." And although **both WHO and UNICEF have offices in Bamako and in all African capitals, they have quite ignored the health needs of childbearing women** including the damage done to women and girls by traditional practices. All this is detailed and documented in **The HOSKEN REPORT,** in the chapters on Mali and the "Conspiracy of Silence."

On my visits to Africa I made it a point to also visit the offices of WHO and UNICEF as well as UNDP (United Nations Development Program). Most of these international offices are located in special compounds in luxurious surroundings - air-conditioned and equipped with the latest facilities. But local women, even midwives, have no access to the men who are in charge, who talk to other men in the health ministries and other government offices. **Most of the WHO and UNICEF representatives I found had never visited a maternity hospital in the countries where they are supposed to serve the health needs of families.** When I brought up the subject of FGM they did not want to talk about it and claimed they could not interfere in cultural practices.

And this attitude by the men in charge, mostly physicians in the case of WHO, has changed little over the years. Due to the pressure of women, WHO and UNICEF headquarters in Geneva and New York, respectively, had to at least pretend that they knew about "this problem" by issuing some press releases and reports. **But these are full of false claims and outright misrepresentations, as I established on my visits to their own representatives in Africa.** It has taken **WIN NEWS** years of constant work to make known the facts about FGM that are so carefully hidden by the men who run these agencies and are royally paid for it. In Mali and most of West Africa, **the absence of any concern or commitment** in these very poor countries to assist and support the families and those most in need - women and children - is especially shocking.

Nowhere else in Africa have I heard the urgent need for change pressed as strongly as in Mali; **nowhere else did I find women so conscious, so critical and so aware of the needs of their own society as the midwives at the Gabriel Toure Hospital:**

> "Not until women have a share in all the decisions will anything change in our society, and change we must. It is not possible to just fight against excision or against polygamy or illiteracy - look what is happening. Women are needed everywhere and men must recognize the true position, worth and contributions of women . . . Without women being involved in decision-making, we shall never get anywhere. **Everything must change and most of all men, who still think that they can own a woman. Polygamy must be abolished. It is an evil institution;** it pits woman against woman and it creates suspicion and hate between children who live under constant pressure and threats."

I asked the midwives about family planning, which was introduced in Mali only a few years ago. Maternities give out contraceptives and teach women about birth control.

> **"But all men are opposed to family planning.** It is a scandal to use contraceptives the men say. What else are women good for but to make children? If a woman is not pregnant, she will run around.
>
> **The men have to be taught, if anything is to change!** Men must be re-educated; they must be made conscious of the importance and the contributions and the real role of women. Women must take part in the decisions in every area and must be actively involved in politics. **The woman is the basis of the state and a stable government.** The whole mentality of men must be changed. A man should have only one wife. At present, a woman who is not married is not respected, so men claim, because they want to dominate women.
>
> A woman has to ask permission of her husband for whatever she does; some men still demand that their wives be veiled; it is a matter of male pride so that only he can see her. He controls everything she does and even what clothes she wears. To change these conditions, you must educate the men; only then will things really begin to change."

The Point G Hospital was built by the French on a hill overlooking Bamako. Unless one has transportation, which most women do not, it is hard to reach this hospital. I went to their maternity, located in a long two-story building with verandas all around on the extensive tree planted grounds. **I talked to the midwife in charge:**

> **"All the women coming to this hospital are excised.** To say 'you are not excised' is a great insult. The women are constantly teased about this; therefore, they continue to do it to their children, mostly out of ignorance of the real consequences.

"A woman who is not operated on is not 'serieuse,' she is not a mature person. Today the operations in Bamako are done by the traditional birth attendants, usually on babies before they are 40 days old. The women cut the babies very quickly; they don't know what they are cutting. Often they do terrible damage."

I had arrived at Point G Hospital early in the morning. As everywhere in Africa, the families of the patients were camped on the grounds alongside the hospital buildings and were just finishing their morning meal. To get to the maternity I had to pass by the nursing school. Most of the trainees there are men, since nursing, as in other Moslem countries, is largely a male profession. The only female trainees are those who will become midwives or are planning to work in maternities.

The maternity at the **Gabriel Toure Hospital also gets many cases of abused and injured women, so the midwives related;** many are pregnant and so badly beaten by their husbands that they have to be hospitalized. **Polygamy, the midwives said, is one reason for wife abuse.** There is great tension and rivalry between the wives in a polygamous family and there are frequent quarrels. The husband then beats all of his wives. A woman, even if she is badly injured by the husband and comes to the hospital, is reluctant to press charges because she is afraid of divorce. Divorce is very frequent; a man can divorce a woman - that is, throw her out - at any time. Women are economically dependent on men. **"We earn our own living," said the midwives, "and we don't accept being beaten."**

"A woman must kneel before her husband to receive chastisement from her husband, who beats her because he loves her" is the popular justification for wife abuse in Mali. It is traditionally claimed that a woman who is beaten and maltreated will produce boys who become great men. **The more a woman suffers, the better are her children, it is said.** And if a woman dies in childbirth, it is believed that she goes to heaven - so the midwives said.

Though most of the Malians are Moslem, limiting the men to four wives at one time, divorce is very frequent and easy for a man. Animists can purchase as many wives as they can afford. **There are no requirements that men have to support their wives nor their children.** Traditionally not only in Mali but in most of Africa women are in charge of all children. That is, not only do they take care of them, **but women in rural areas where most families live have to grow the food for all their children, and they have to feed the men as well.** All subsistence farming is done by women which is unpaid and used to sustain the families. Cash crops are grown by men, who therefore get governmental support and services from agricultural agents, but women do not.

In 1991, the story of Aminata, a young woman from Mali who fled to Paris to escape being excised, became a typical media sensation and was first exploited all over France. Aminata was finally flown to the US by the National Organization for Women (NOW) to be featured at an international conference in Washington, D.C., where she was made to speak. But she did not understand or speak a word of English. **While addressing hundreds of women in a huge hall to tell her sad story she predictably lost her composure. No one could understand a word she said in West African French.**

Aminata was born in a village near Sikasso in the southeastern part of Mali. When it came time to get married - her marriage had been arranged years ago by her father - she first had to be excised, as tradition demands. It is the custom where her family lives to excise all girls just before they are married, usually in their early teens - and none can escape.

Aminata's best friend had died from excision a few weeks earlier, after suffering terribly for days. Therefore Aminata refused to undergo this torture after returning home from Bamako, where she went to school. Her father insisted, and called in the Marabout, the local Moslem leader, to persuade her. But she still refused and went back to Bamako. Fortunately for Aminata, she had made friends there with an airline attendant who arranged for her to fly to Paris.

At first, the French Government would not allow her to stay as she did not have refugee status, but finally an exception was made in her case. **Aminata found many supporters in her plight, becoming a cause celebre in Paris** for a while. With education and new friends she was able to look forward to a better life than what was prescribed for her by her father - to be one of several mutilated wives of a villager in a remote area of Mali, working from dawn to dusk to feed her many children.

It is Aminata's mother who is the real victim of this situation, however, but no one anywhere speaks for her. Though she was the senior wife she was thrown out of their house by her husband, who kept all her children, leaving her with nothing at all. In the view of the men who run this society, it is the mother who is always blamed if a daughter does something "wrong."

Meanwhile, in this country, NOW had enlisted magazines and tabloids to cover the story as well as television networks for live interviews. But since Aminata could not speak on TV the networks refused, and the ambitious media plans of NOW to exploit Aminata's visit failed.

As the largest women's organization of the US, the NOW national management should have had better judgment than to try to exhibit a young woman from a Malian village to gain publicity. Aminata went back to France, and by now her story is quite forgotten, as most media exploits usually are. NOW's publicity stunt did nothing at all to change the situation for girls and women in Mali, or anywhere else in Africa.

The French Government continues to refuse to recognize FGM as a reason for granting political asylum, which Aminata's lawyer tried to achieve - in vain - to set a precedent. Other countries, Canada, for instance, have granted women refugee status for persecution on gender grounds. The US is now considering to grant women asylum on gender grounds, and recently some cases were heard. Last year, a Nigerian woman and her young daughters, who were at risk of undergoing FGM if they returned to Nigeria, were allowed to stay in the US.

In African towns and capitals one can find many young women who escape from the brutalities of traditional village life. Cut off from all family support and unable to earn a living for lack of education, they have no choice but to become prostitutes. The status of a daughter in Mali who is repudiated by her family in a country that recognizes no independent life for women outside the family, means that **no one will marry her or employ her, and she is cut off from all social and community life**. She is no longer regarded as a Moslem, as local Moslem leaders claim that excision is a religious requirement. This claim is made by the Moslem leaders all over West Africa though it is not in the Koran. But in traditional communities religious leaders are all powerful.

Assitan Diallo wrote in her thesis at the Teacher's College in Bamako about the traditions still practiced by the Bambara, the largest ethnic group of Mali, all of whom excise their daughters just before marriage. However, in Bamako proper, the operations now are done on ever younger girls and most of the rituals are omitted.

> "Excision at the Bambara takes place in the cool season (November/February). Women, according to Islamic beliefs, are considered 'impure' unless excised. When Mali was converted to Islam, the Bambara population already practiced excision, in order to confirm each individual's sex and make him/her acceptable in society. It is believed that the clitoris represents the male element in a young girl, while the prepuce represents femininity for a boy.
>
> Therefore, to become a fully accepted member of adult society, both have to be removed at the initiation ceremony. It is also believed traditionally by the Bambara that the clitoris and prepuce are the seat of an evil spirit called 'Wanzo,' and this Wanzo prevents its possessor from having a union with a member of the opposite sex; therefore, they must be removed."

While visiting Bamako recently I was invited to a meeting on the outskirts of the city with local women, arranged by the Centre Djoliba, a Catholic organization which runs various education programs. Some years ago I had been contacted by one of their sisters, a woman from the Netherlands, who taught there and asked for our **Childbirth Picture Books with the Additions to Prevent Excision and Infibulation**. Since then I have been regularly sending them many hundreds of the French books to use for teaching and distributing to local groups.

Mme. Sidibe Kadidia coordinates some women's programs for the Centre Djoliba and is from northern Mali where, she told me, FGM is not practiced. I went along to one of their neighborhood women's meeting on the outskirts of Bamako where excision was discussed. The meeting took place on the empty ground floor of a house with a large porch. The room was packed with women of all ages who spoke Bambara and some French; **a noisy discussion had already started. Many women strongly defended excision:**

> "A woman has to be excised to be a woman - otherwise she is like a man. . . It is necessary to do to have children though the Koran does not say so. . . It is done because the clitoris is dirty. . . It is necessary for health. . . The clitoris closes the vagina when the woman has sex with her husband, so it has to be cut off . . . The clitoris is dangerous, it can kill a baby during birth. . . It is done so that girls keep their virginity. . . If the girl is not operated, she will run after men, that is why it is done. . . Now it is done on little girls, as it is necessary to be healthy. . ."

These are but some of the reasons given by the women. **It is the caste of the forgeron - the blacksmith caste - who traditionally do the operations in Mali.** The wives of the blacksmiths are the excisors, since they have access to sharp metal tools. This occupation is hereditary, as the caste system still prevails in Mali today. Infibulation was also discussed. "It is done by closing the legs of the girls after excision and tying them together - then a scar forms and closes the vagina, showing that the girl is 'intact.'"

Next, the discussion turned to where excision comes from and how it started. "It goes back to ancient times," the women said. "Ibrahim's first wife demanded that his second wife, whom he took to have children, must be excised because she was jealous. Thereafter, excision was practiced."

The women, especially the older, very vocal ones, had plenty of time to assert their beliefs and influence the younger ones. Then a nurse who had come with us explained the damage done and the difficulties that often result in childbirth due to the scars. "Did you not have problems?" she asked the women, all of whom were excised. Some readily admitted that they had encountered problems.

Finally, Mme. Sidibe stepped forward to provide some facts. By then, many women had left and others had joined the meeting. A flannel flip chart was used to show the female genital organs **and to visually demonstrate what happens as a result of excision and why life-threatening bleeding occurs.** The nurse who had come with us explained the medical facts in detail and used a large plastic model, which was donated to the program by the Inter- African Committee, to demonstrate the physical results of excision. Many questions were answered by showing and demonstrating what happens with the anatomic model, which was well understood by the women, but by that time, unfortunately, the older pro-excision leaders had left.

On the way back, Mme. Sidibe explained it was important to give women the opportunity to voice their ideas. But since no presentation was made at the beginning to provide any facts, the most vocal and opinionated women took over, promoting FGM and their traditional views. No one else, least of all the younger women who might have had other ideas, had a chance to be heard. Unless a meeting, especially on such a controversial subject, provides the facts and objectives at the beginning - to teach about health and explain the dangers of excision - the traditionalists take over as happened here.

By the time the nurse had had a chance to speak and the model was shown demonstrating the damage done by FGM, the women who had strongly supported FGM had left. They were the leaders and had won the day in their own community. To teach about change requires a persuasive, well-planned program rather than offering participants an opportunity to talk; because what usually happens is that those who affirm the status quo take over.

The advantage of the Childbirth Picture Books with the Additions on Excision and Infibulation is that they can be handed out and looked at in privacy after a meeting by each participant. For teachers they include a complete discussion guide that involves all participants from the start. The books have also been widely used for self teaching, with no presenter needed, since the pictures are quite simple and explicit, showing the basic facts about reproduction and the damage done by FGM: they are effective even for those who cannot read, and that is certainly the vast majority in Mali and most of West Africa.

The Childbirth Picture Books in French are widely distributed in Mali, especially to the midwifery school. Books can be readily distributed to circulate throughout the community so that men can also be reached, which is most important as men make most of the decisions and stay away from women's meetings. **Books furthermore can reach remote areas and can be shared by many people who cannot come to meetings: it is possible to reach many more people with printed information that is persuasive since it can be looked at again and again and discussed with others in the community.**

It is difficult to establish whether or not attitudes are changing in this very conservative Moslem country. One change that has been widely reported for sometime is that, for instance, in Bamako FGM is no longer practiced as a puberty rite as tradition requires and which still continues in rural areas - it is now done on ever younger children. **The midwives at the Gabriel Toure Hospital reported that an excisor works right in the hospital to operate on newborn babies; they claimed this was much better so that if any problems should arise a doctor on the premises can take care of them.**

To mutilate ever younger children is the trend not only in Bamako but in urban areas everywhere in Africa. Traditional rituals are being discarded, but the operations continue which demonstrate their real purpose: sexual castration of women to affirm control and domination by men. **At the same time, more and more trained health workers - both women and men - are doing the mutilations for money, quite aside from physicians.**

There are many Malian immigrants living in Paris; ostensibly men go to France to work but some stay there for years and bring their wives. Since many have children, excision has become a problem as it is against French law. Three little girls of Malian immigrants recently bled to death as a result of excision. **Their mutilations were done by excisors brought to France from Mali for that purpose, and one was operated on by the father with a pen knife.**

Most of the immigrant women are illiterate, but since all mothers in France are required to bring their babies for check-ups and shots to baby clinics this offered an opportunity to talk to the mothers, warning them that excision is prohibited and teaching them why. The women coming to the health centers with their children are encouraged to tell their stories. **A woman from Mali, who has lived in France for two years, tells her story:**

"I was operated at sunrise, after a festival the day before. My mother had told me that I must not cry and not even move to preserve the honor of the family, though it will hurt. After the operation, I must dance to express my happiness. The excisor, the wife of a blacksmith, would do the operation and I should sit down and open my legs. The pain was absolutely dreadful but I did my best to control myself out of respect for my family.

In the Bambara language, to excise means 'to sit on a knife.' This indicates that the participation of the girl in her excision is required. In the language of the Saracole, to excise means 'to give her the right to pray' because many believe that a woman who is not excised cannot properly perform her ablutions. After she is purified by her excision, a girl can pray to God.

When my daughters were born, at first I didn't want to have them excised. But in my country one says many bad things about girls who are not excised. One says they will be ugly and sterile, and they cannot control their sexuality. So I had them excised a short time after they were born so that at least they would not remember the pain. I think if I had been older, I would have had the strength to resist because today, I know all that one says about excision in my country is entirely wrong. Religion does not require it and it is very dangerous. Excision is also an offense against women's rights. For all these reasons, I have decided to work against excision. It is important to stress the issue of their rights to African women

When I came to France, I was invited by the African families in my neighborhood, and I invited them back to my house, as is the custom. The women stick together to help each other and we talk about our children, our husbands, and about the strange land in which we now live. The first step towards a solution is to talk about it. **The women are now discussing excision, they need more information. The time has come to organize meetings with the help of the clinics where we take our children.**"

BURKINA FASO

Burkina Faso is one of the poorest countries in the world, and most of the population depends on subsistence farming. Recent droughts have worsened the situation as the Sahara Desert steadily moves south all over West Africa, eating up more and more arable land. Many men leave, trying to find paid employment in neighboring countries.

The plight of women in this very traditional society is devastating. Work is divided according to gender; women do some of the hardest labor including most of the subsistence farming to support their children and to feed all members of the household. But according to deeply rooted tradition, all land belongs to men, women own nothing. Girls without exception are excised before marriage in drastic ways with often lifelong damage to their health and constant pain as a result.

The official literacy figures say 27 percent - which means probably fewer than 12 percent of women can read, and those are usually concentrated in or around the capital or the few towns. As a neglected region of the French colonial administration of West Africa the education and health of women in Burkina Faso were never a concern in Upper Volta, the name of the country until 1983. As elsewhere in West Africa, the French administration trained a small elite group of men to work for them and a few women to run their households, French-style, but most of the country pursued its traditional ways.

The health statistics are dismal. Infant and maternal mortality are among the highest in the world. Until a few years ago women were part of the property inherited by men. Despite some very recent laws which are only beginning to be implemented in the capital, this situation no doubt continues in rural areas where hardly anyone can read.

The tradition-bound lives of women in Burkina Faso, which are now being changed by the country's leadership, should disabuse those still persuaded by politicians and anthropologists that tradition must be preserved. Who has not heard politicians in Africa admonish women from a rostrum to "keep and preserve our hallowed traditions"? This really means go back to the kitchen and keep out of politics; we don't want you here. **Custom and tradition, not only in Africa but all over the world, are used as excuses to continue to exclude women from politics, education and decision-making to preserve patriarchal control and a host of damaging violent practices to restrict women's lives.**

The leadership of Burkina Faso is setting an example for all of Africa. After determining that the country needs to change to improve the living conditions of its people mired in deep poverty, both men and women are working hard to improve living conditions, which means abolishing the terribly damaging customs and traditions that have restricted development and excluded half the population - women - from taking control over their own lives. More and more people realize that the younger generation must be educated and freed from traditional restrictions to compete in today's world and improve living conditions for the future of their own society. In no other country has the necessity for change been so widely recognized by the leadership and government.

What are these traditional practices? The most pervasive one is FGM, which is practiced all over the country, as described by a woman physician of Burkina Faso:

> "The age at which excision is performed varies, but the girls are accepted for the operation as soon as they begin to grow pubic hair. No girl may refuse. The medicine man of the village determines the date and the place of the operation - usually an area outside the village, early in the morning. In order to prevent 'accidents,' certain rites must be followed and sacrifices (chickens and goats, for instance) are made, and banishments against evil spirits are pronounced.

> The excisor digs a hole in the ground over which each girl must sit to be operated on. The girls are told they must not cry because this can cause the death of their mothers. The operation takes place with many women 'helpers' who shout as loud as they can to cover up the screams of the victims. After the operation, the wound is washed with hot water and soap and then a salve of clay or cinders and butter is directly applied to stop the bleeding. The evening after the excision, the operator applies a liquid made with several plants, and this treatment is repeated on the following days. These dressings of dirt and cinders cannot stop the bleeding, and they greatly increase the chances of infection.

When some girls die, either from hemorrhage or infection, this is blamed on fate or it is said that certain customs have not been properly observed. But it is never the responsibility of the operator.

The psychological consequences of the operations represent the most horrible ordeal of each girl's young life, that they are forced to suffer under the threat of even worse punishments. No matter at what age the operation is performed, due to the traumatization of the sexual area most or all sexual pleasure of the woman is eradicated. It also often happens that all sexual intercourse becomes very painful.

Every woman remembers the acute pain of the operation throughout her life, and this memory is evoked with each sexual intercourse. Permanent psychosis may result from such a torturous sex life.

Young brides, after suffering the repeated pains of intercourse, hope to be free of this torment when they become pregnant. However, the birth process often creates worse problems and even greater agonies that some women are unable to face. Many become depressed and psychotic; some lose their minds. There are also many suicide attempts caused by these problems they are unable to escape."

A woman working for the health department, who visits many remote areas, reports what she has observed:

"The operation consists of an incision made the length of the small lips up to the clitoris with the special knife of the excisor. A piece of wire is then hooked into the clitoris to pull it out completely and cut it off at its root. The girl is then forced to get up and made to jump twice over the hole which is full of blood and the pieces of flesh cut out of the girls. Afterward each girl is made to sit down and watch the others while they are operated on. The girls must then eat some millet while various ceremonies are performed. Then they are taken to a house where a woman applies some ointment made of cinders and butter to their wounds."

When I first visited Ouagadougou I went to the maternity of the Yalgado Hospital to talk to Dr. Joseph Kabore, who had invited me to come and see him there early in the morning. The maternity is in a separate building. The relatives of the patients, who are often a long way from home, had camped on the grounds and were just waking up. Dr. Kabore had invited me to ask him any questions when a midwife came to call him to the delivery room; he asked me to come along. **A very young woman had been brought in with an enormous belly, ready to deliver what was obviously her first child. She was on a gurney, completely naked, and the midwife pointed to the woman's vagina, which was completely closed.** There was no way for the baby to come out without major surgery. She evidently must have conceived through a tiny opening, which happens quite often, so medical reports confirm.

Women's organizations in Burkina Faso have tried for years to organize campaigns against these mutilations, but they were rebuffed until recently. In the 1970's, a radio program was organized by **the national women's organization under the leadership of Alice Tiendrebeogo** and with the help of Dr. Kabore and other leaders. But the reaction from the Moslem leaders was so negative that they had to stop. Tiendrebeogo also attended the WHO seminar in Khartoum in 1979, but it took nearly another decade until the present campaign was organized.

This campaign, supported by the government, formally started in May 1988 with a national seminar on "Traditional Practices Affecting the Health of Women: The Case of Excision and Proposals for Elimination" in Ouagadougou. It was sponsored by Action Sociale, a ministry of the government that was then headed by Tiendrebeogo, who had been working to stop FGM for nearly 20 years and finally had gained public support.

The seminar, held in three local languages and French, was designed to raise the consciousness of the people and its leaders and to develop a strategy to stop FGM. This national meeting was held just a few weeks before the memorable international conference held in Mogadishu, in June 1988, to gain support for the government-sponsored national campaign of Somalia run by the SWDO (Somali Women's Democratic Organization) and AIDoS (Italian Organization of Women in Development) and financed by the Italian Government.

But the campaign in Burkina Faso does not have the support that Somalia had from Italy and Italian women; the French Government has ignored initiatives to eradicate damaging traditions, and French women's organizations have shown little interest in the needs of women in Africa, though some sophisticated African women live in Paris and are often prominently featured by the French fashion world.

The specific strategies of this campaign are detailed in the "Case History of Burkina Faso" in **The HOSKEN REPORT and WIN NEWS**. The campaign strives to:

> "... involve everyone, women and men, grandparents, and all other family members, to start discussions in villages and urban centers. Women especially must make the men of their families aware of the suffering involved."

Specific strategies include: the mobilization of resources for the campaign; legislation or specific measures to stop excision; organization of provincial committees; invitations to religious authorities to join the campaign; development of information and education programs and materials; research studies where needed; introduction of the subject in national education programs and schools; involvement of all media, and much more.

The discussion of the damage done by FGM has been going on for years, at least in Ouagadougou, where health services are available to those in the government. Some families choose "the modern way" to excise their daughters, as a woman reports:

> "Under the influence of 'development,' excision continues to be practiced but in an antiseptic environment in clinics and hospitals. The instruments are sterilized, and after the operation the wound is dressed according to modern methods. Anti-tetanus injections are given and the parents make the girls take antibiotics. There is no ritual of any kind, and no mystery surrounds this sexual castration operation."

For fathers, the incentive clearly is the brideprice, which in Burkina Faso - as everywhere else in Africa - is a great economic inducement to see to it that their daughters are mutilated. Fathers do not want to lose the girls as the brideprice would also be lost. Hence they choose the medical way even if it costs more. It is the same now in all major towns in Africa. This is known to WHO, as they have local representatives in all African capitals, and to internationally financed **health and population programs, which have failed to take preventive actions even in their program areas. Imported antibiotics and tools are now used to mutilate girls - as I have pointed out in Congressional testimonies since 1980.**

In a country where most of the population is illiterate it is not easy to reach the people, let alone their hearts and minds. Initiatives for change until recently have been limited to the capital and a few towns. Therefore in the autumn of 1989, the 72-minute film **"My Daughter Will Not Be Excised" was launched in Ouagadougou by the Minister of Information and Culture together with the Secretary of State of Action Sociale, Alice Tiendrebeogo.** The film was shot in the rural areas of Burkina Faso with mostly local people and took two years to make. It is the story of a traditional village family; one of their sons is sent to school and finally studies medicine. He becomes a physician, and with his own family regularly visits his parents in the village. He refuses to have his teen-age daughter operated though this is against the wishes of his father and the entire family.

This drama, with which most rural people can identify (the girl is rescued at the last minute from a forced excision), draws the people who see it into the action. **The film is shown by the National Committee on the Eradication of Excision all over the country and is used for creating awareness of the physical, social and economic consequences of the mutilations, raising questions among the audience about the problems in their own communities.** The film is used as a vehicle for change, to start the discussion session at meetings arranged by the committee, and to initiate health education.

This unique approach may also be useful in other African countries where similar conditions exist. Yet this campaign, despite the fact that it is the only one in Africa that has not only governmental support but is run by the Government, does not have the necessary international financing and technical assistance that is so very important and which was available in Somalia. A campaign report, which also includes a five-year plan and budget, outlines visits of the committee to communities all over the country to bring local people together and show the film. Unfortunately, it also includes many references that some scheduled meetings had to be canceled for lack of money.

The French edition of the **Childbirth Picture Books with the Additions to Prevent Excision** are widely used all over the country. **WIN NEWS** has sent hundreds each year to the midwifery school and the Ministry of Health. Each time I visited Burkina Faso I discussed the use and distribution of these books with pertinent local decision makers; an offer was made by **WIN NEWS** to send as many to the campaign as needed.

At the Inter-African Committee conference in Addis Ababa in April 1994, the first lady of the country, Mme. Chantal Compaore, wife of the president of Burkina Faso, came to participate in the conference and to lend her country's official support. She spoke about the national campaign and described how the education and sensitizing initiatives are carried on all over the country, with film showings, posters, leaflets, talks, discussions and all available media support as well as the participation of all government ministries.

On my last visit to Burkina Faso I went again to the maternity of the Yalgado Hospital to talk to some of the midwives. **Because of the World Bank/International Monetary Fund austerity imposed on the government, which has resulted in drastic reductions of all services, the hospital is desperately short of equipment and medicines of all kinds.** Maternity services are cut most of all, and that is the same in all African countries, as women lack all political power and influence. I showed the **Childbirth Picture Books** to Mme. Traore, one of the midwives at the hospital, and we agreed to meet again after her work was finished. This is what she told me:

> "Practically all the women coming to the hospital are excised, but now more and more women are coming to seek help at the hospital, while only a few years ago they mainly went to the traditional birth attendants and healers. As you saw at the hospital there are long lines of people waiting to see a doctor or nurse, and this goes on every day, we cannot keep up with even the most urgent needs. Most of the time we have not enough medicines and have to send many to the pharmacy in town to buy what they need, but that is too expensive for many."

Mme. Traore works as a midwife at the hospital. As a government employee - health care is a government responsibility - she has her own income. She told me that since her husband died she alone has to support her three children, ages 12, 10 and 8:

> "My husband worked for the government and was killed a year ago in a car accident while on the job. I am supposed to get insurance and a pension, but his family took all his papers and documents, then they threw me and the children out of the house. His relatives took the house and all we owned when I turned down their decision that I was to be given to one of his brothers - this is the tradition here. They made life impossible for me. I had to go to live with my family which is headed by my younger brother, who is afraid to stand up against the powerful elders of my husband's family. If I tried to oppose them it would not be regarded well. I don't know how I shall pay the school fees for the children, besides everything else."

Though legislation was passed recently to give widows some rights, it evidently is not implemented even in the capital. Social pressure is too great, women have no way to defend themselves against the patriarchal family heads who are only interested in taking women's property. Mme. Traore is Catholic, but the priest of her parish did not help.

Finally, there is the story of a woman from Burkina Faso who had gone with her husband to France where they lived for more than 10 years. She went home to visit her mother and family with her three daughters whom they had never seen. After she arrived, her mother-in-law questioned her about the children. **When her mother-in-law learned that they were not operated she got very upset and left:**

> "I explained that we had decided they would not be excised as several girls we knew had died. A few days later two men from my husband's family came to tell me that a letter from him had arrived, that I must immediately go to live with his mother. But I grew suspicious and refused, because she had insisted my girls must be excised. I realized that I had better leave and rented a car to go to the town. But my brother, whom I had asked to drive us, refused. Fortunately I found someone else as I had **some money from my husband and we drove straight to the nearest airport to get** a connecting flight to Paris. My in-laws pursued me all the way to the airport. I shall never go back to Africa until my daughters are grown up and married."

Mariam, who lives in a small town north of Ouagadougou, just delivered her third child and first daughter, though she is only 20. Girls are married very young in her community; the brideprice is a great incentive for fathers to arrange marriages early. **"Shall I cut her now?"** the midwife asks the mother. She expects to get an extra payment for this "service." **"No, you cannot; my husband forbids it."**

Mariam herself was excised when she was a small child. This was quite unusual as where her family lived group initiations were the rule. Young girls were excised and initiated just before they were married in their early teens. But her father had been to school in a nearby small town and was taught to read and write and also worked at the local hospital where he learned about many health problems. **He had all his daughters excised early rather than as teenagers, as is the custom. He knew he could not get them married unless they were excised.** But several teenagers, the daughters of friends, had problems when they were initiated: some girls bled to death as no one could stop it. The doctor who visited the health center from time to time and whom the father asked said excision was less dangerous to do when the girls are still very young. **Mariam therefore was operated on as a small child. She tells her story:**

"Of course I remember everything: I had no idea what was happening when my mother called me early one morning to the backyard and said the midwife from a nearby village was waiting for me and my sister. I knew that the older girls went together outside the village to a special place to be initiated, and they stayed there for some time; when they came back they were married immediately with much celebration and feasting. But I did not know what happened at that special place; we were not allowed to go there.

But I was only 5 when the midwife and her helper cut me and my sister while her helpers held us down. I was terrified. We were told we must not cry, but that was impossible; it hurt too much. Afterwards the wound kept on hurting for weeks; we could not walk for days; urination continued to burn for a long time. I thought I would never get well again, and cried and cried. I asked why the midwife did this to us; what had we done to be punished in this dreadful way. My mother said it had to be done or no man would ever want to marry us; it was better to do it when we were little by a midwife because if we waited to do it later with the other girls it would be much worse. The excisor in our village had many accidents lately as she was getting very old.

Much later, after I was sent to school when we moved into a nearby town, I finally found out what had been done to me and that **all the other girls in school were also operated. It was necessary to have children, they said.** And not to have children was the worst thing that could happen to anyone. My father arranged my marriage to a man from a family in the same town, which is fortunate as I sometimes can go to see my mother. The man to whom I am married already had a wife and when I moved there I had to help her with her children and all the work. But I could read, as I had gone to school for three years before I was married, and so I went to the market to sell what we grew and could not eat. In the market I talked to other women and there were some people who talked about how to take care of children, what to feed them and what to do when they were ill.

One woman said they should not be excised because it is dangerous; she said it should be stopped, that it was not necessary to do to have children. Quite a few people came to listen and asked her questions. I told my husband what she said; he had also heard her speak. He asked the people at the clinic. **They all said it is bad and should not be done because it may be dangerous and that many women have problems in childbirth as a result.**

Yes, with my first child I was in labor for many hours, but they said it is the first one and that is always hard. I bled a lot and was very sore; the woman in the market had said that childbirth difficulties are caused by the operations. But I had been cut by the midwife when I was still little, **so why would it hurt me many years later when I had my first child?** Still, my husband says he does not want to have his daughters excised.

My co-wife said her first daughter, who is 13, needs to be initiated now. But he told her no; he is very opposed to it. And since she has no money and he won't pay for it, she can't get it done. They don't do it here in our town; the girl would have to be sent to her grandmother in the village, but he forbade it. **He said that the families in our town don't want to spend money for wives who are excised** for their sons, because the wives may die in childbirth or be sick and unable to work, and they would spend the brideprice for nothing. The doctor at the clinic is also against it. **So I will not have my daughter excised."**

Awa does not know how old she is. Her face is very sad, her head bent down and her emaciated body is covered by rags. I saw her sitting by herself at the dusty edge of the road, holding onto a long stick near the many bicycles parked there by market visitors. Rows of booths with narrow pathways in between covered the whole market square. One of the big market women came out of the back of her booth and gave her an old tin plate with some scraps of food which Awa eagerly stuffed into her mouth.

I asked the woman, after buying some of her wares, about her gesture of kindness that I had observed and if she knew the sad, abandoned waif by the side of the road.

"Her name is Awa and she is the oldest daughter of my mother's co-wife. We had to take her in as her husband threw her out because she is incontinent. She is not so old, but she just looks that way. We let her sleep near the house and she follows me to market everyday; but no one can stand being near her because she smells.

She was married right after her initiation and excision and had a child right away, though she was still very young. The baby was born dead, after they finally took her to the clinic after two days, and she nearly died herself; she was very weak from bleeding so much. **The midwives at the clinic said she would have to go to the hospital in the capital to have an operation, but that costs a lot.**

Her husband now has two other wives to do the work and have his children. She was starving when she came back to us so we have to feed her; but she cannot do much work as she can hardly walk and no one has any use for her. The operation she needs is very expensive; we have no money and there is no one to take her to the hospital, which is far away."

Amna Coulibaly is very distraught. She is a big, strong woman, sure of herself and her opinions and always ready to smile as well as argue. But lately she has not been herself. Finally, she confided in her best friend, who had asked her again and again why she was so upset. **In tears she finally told her story:**

"My husband just took another wife. This is the third one and she is so much younger and is no help at all in the house. The second one I finally got rid of; she was lazy and did not know anything but to flatter men. She left saying she could not live in a household with me. I was glad to be rid of her. I had tried for a year to get her to go, and I was really glad when I succeeded. But now he took another one; I don't know where he got the money, I did not know anything about it. **But the worst thing is she is not even excised.**

One day he brought her to our house and told me she was here to stay! He has been with her ever since and has ignored me completely. **I am his first wife; I have run his house and have borne him four children. Why does he want another one who is not even a proper woman because she is not excised, and that is a shame!**

What can I do; he prefers her. When I said she was not excised and that is a disgrace for our whole family he told me he likes it that way. He said he prefers to be with her because she is not cut. **What can I do, I am desperate. Now he rejects me, saying I am excised!** What will become of my children?

We were proud to be initiated and excised, the girls who were not were laughed at and teased, and no man would even look at them. **Everyone knows to be a real woman you have to be initiated or no man will pay the brideprice. So we suffered all this pain and we were proud of it. And now my own husband turns me down!"**

SIERRA LEONE

In Sierra Leone, a very small country of less than 4 million people, FGM is practiced by the secret women's societies called Bundu. Only the Creoles, who are 2 percent of the population and whose ancestors were repatriated former slaves, do not practice FGM; they face discrimination as a result. Most of the Creoles live in Freetown, the capital.

These secret and often powerful women's societies traditionally promoted women and provided the political basis for women chiefs. Their counterpart, the secret societies of men, called Porro, in turn support the male chiefs who ruled the country. But now, modernization and development with contemporary political structures and outside influences have caused the traditional system to lose much of its influence. As a reaction, the traditionalists are rejecting all modernization. Still, the initiations continue, surrounded by magic and carried out in special areas outside each villages. These initiations include excision laced with all kinds of magic and done as group ceremony; often the presiding matron, who knows nothing about anatomy, makes additional cuts into the vagina that result in terrible wounds. Many girls bleed to death even if they are taken to a clinic, which is difficult in rural areas where roads and transportation are very poor.

Since the secret women's societies are steeped in mystery they attract the young girls who often are eager to participate in the initiations, which make them for once the center of attention - they also get presents and new clothes. **As all members are sworn to secrecy the girls have no idea what awaits them, and are afraid of the magic powers of the women who conduct the ceremonies.** Only in Liberia, the neighbor of Sierra Leone, a similar system of secret societies exists, with devastating results for both the health of women and the development of the country. Sierra Leone is beset with economic problems; unable to feed itself the country now has to import food while in the past it produced a surplus.

Traditionally women paramount chiefs were admired figures, but today an education is much more important than the magic of secret rites, which still continue in the rural areas where modern education has not reached. Literacy, according to official statistics, is about 15 percent for both men and women, which means in this society that more than 90 percent of women can neither read nor write.

It is forbidden to all Bundu members to tell what happens in the secret bush where initiations are conducted and where the girls of each area are mutilated as a group. For a long time the real facts of the mutilations were concealed, including the terrible health damage done to girls and women who were not allowed to tell what happened to them under threat of the Bundu matron. Each group of girls had to stay in the Bundu bush under the watchful eyes of the Bundu chief and her helpers, until they healed or died. **But the death of a daughter in the secret bush was never blamed on the matron or the rituals conducted there, but it was, and still is, ascribed to evil spirits,** which seem especially plentiful and damaging all over Sierra Leone, so most of its inhabitants state. Many people firmly believe that magic powers of all kinds regulate their lives.

Only recently, after women began to seek help in modern health facilities rather than from traditional healers and midwives, has the real damage become apparent. For instance, Dr. Olayinka Koso-Thomas, a physician who has worked for years for the health ministry and now has a private clinic for women, conducted a research study on this subject. She found that 95 percent of women surveyed suffered from obstructed labor (as compared to 5 percent of women who are not excised). More than 85 percent of the young girls who are excised need medical attention afterwards, but only less than half actually get help.

Dr. Koso-Thomas points out that quite aside from the terrible damage to women's health and productiveness the costs of treating girls and women are staggering. These costs make up a significant portion of the country's health budget. Dr. Koso-Thomas states:

> "It has now come to the nation as a rude shock that this practice is reducing the proportion of young fertile females in the population who could contribute to the developing society. A population consisting of so large a proportion of unhealthy women can never make the progress expected of it towards economic and social development. Modern Sierra Leone needs all the hands she can mobilize. Women must contribute to the fullest extent and with a healthy, sound body and mind. . ."

Both Temne and Mende, the two dominant ethnic groups, initiate their daughters - that is, they are excised by the secret societies. Following that they are immediately married. Polygamy is widely practiced, and important men in the rural areas can purchase an unlimited number of wives. Very young girls are often forced to leave school to join the rural household of a man as another wife, adding to his agricultural labor force.

A young woman student at Fourah-Bay College in Freetown, the best-known institution of higher learning in anglophone West Africa, states:

> "Before acquiring an education, I was a great admirer of the Bundu society. At one time, before my relatives could afford the expenses to have me initiated, I almost ran into the bush when I heard all the beautiful singing there. In which case I would have been initiated immediately. Yes, I was very proud of one day becoming a member of the society. I did not then realize the danger to health incurred by having the clitoris cut out without surgical precautions.
>
> When I came to college . . . I learned that this operation had several bad effects which can complicate childbirth. The immediate effect is sometimes so dangerous as to be fatal. When I was initiated, one of the girls almost bled to death. I see no reason why women should join this society, and one day I was bold enough to tell my mother that if they waited until I got to secondary school, before they decided to have me initiated, I would never have joined. I have sworn that none of my daughters will suffer what I had to suffer due to ignorance.
>
> Western education has almost eradicated the practice of forcing women, especially the Creole women, to join the society. The illiterate members of the Bundu society sometimes pick a quarrel deliberately with those who are against this evil practice, and when they berate the practice, they are dragged into the Bundu bush and initiated by force. . . After such an incident the Bundu women were sent to prison and the initiation rites and especially the operation, which are supposed to be secret, were exposed in the local newspaper."

The **"Case History on Sierra Leone"** of **The HOSKEN REPORT** provides a detailed description of a traditional initiation of girls in the Bundu bush. Economic incentives strongly support the continuation of FGM; the average fee paid to the Bundu matron represents a substantial expense for each family and provides a large income for the operators, the Bundu matrons, who want to continue this trade and reject all change.

Dr. Koso-Thomas, whose research and survey is cited above, wrote a book on a strategy for eradication of FGM in Sierra Leone, the first such national plan for any African country.* **The economics of this plan should be convincing to every government as the plan would practically pay for itself within 20 years in terms of health care costs saved,** quite aside from enhancing the economic contributions of women, many of whom lose much work time because of health problems due to the damaging results of FGM. The Government, the largest employer, has to pay for this as well as for medical care.

The plan of Dr. Koso-Thomas, a step-by-step program over a 20-year period, involves the entire country and population and proceeds in stages. It also includes training for excisors to make a living in other ways, as they enjoy a special status in each community. A Health Care Plan to take care of women who have been excised as girls is part of the plan as they face health problems for the rest of their lives. A Health Education Program teaches about reproduction, child care, nutrition and more. A comprehensive budget accompanies the plan which shows that it will be amortized over the life of the plan and supported from the savings of health care costs for taking care of the mutilated girls, who increasingly come to government clinics seeking help after they are excised.

Dr. Koso-Thomas is the regional director of the Inter-African Committee and has participated and organized many regional and local meetings. She has used many of the **Childbirth Picture Books** sent by **WIN NEWS** for her local meetings and continues to distribute them all over the country.

---

*Olayinka Koso-Thomas, M.D., M.P.H. **Circumcision of Women: A Strategy for Eradication,** Zed Books Ltd., 57 Caledonian Road, London, N1 9BU, UK (1987).

In Freetown, I went to the midwifery school in the largest maternity hospital, which is well equipped compared to the terrible conditions that I had observed in Mali and Burkina Faso, both francophone countries. The trained midwives have to deal with all the problems in childbirth that result from FGM, including obstructed labor. But it is a formidable task to communicate these facts to the families and even to community health workers who are not trained in midwifery.

The relationship between the mutilations, which are often inflicted years before childbirth, and the problems in delivery, such as obstructed labor, is not understood by most people, nor is hemorrhaging after the operation attributed to the cutting. People know that only few girls die from the operation nor do all women have problems in childbirth. Therefore in Sierra Leone the problems are attributed to evil spirits, to witchcraft and all kinds of supernatural powers that lurk everywhere and are a constant danger, so people believe.

How can the facts be explained to people who are illiterate, therefore unable to relate cause and effect and unaccustomed to using a rational approach? Because literacy is so low, the **Childbirth Picture Book (CBPB), which tells the whole story of reproduction in pictures, has been especially successful in the rural areas of Sierra Leone. From no other country has WIN NEWS received as many requests for more books.**

Included in the back of each book, together with the **Addition to Prevent Excision,** is an insert addressed to the reader to send **WIN NEWS a note promising not to have his/her daughter operated - now that they have learned about the problems that result. In return, more books will be sent to anyone who responds.** I began some seven years ago to enclose this insert with all books that include the Additions to Prevent Excision or Infibulation; it was an instant success. **WIN NEWS** has been getting hundreds of letters from the grass-roots level by both women and men from all over Africa where the books are distributed. They circulate throughout many communities judging from the letters that arrive with both promises to stop the operations and requests for more books. (See Appendix.)

The largest response has been from Sierra Leone, mostly from local people in the interior rather than from Freetown. But letters also come from all other countries where the **CBPBs** with Additions are sent. The books circulate from person to person in many communities. These letters are from health workers, schoolteachers, midwives, nurses, students, community leaders, local clinics, schools and various local groups. **Many people write about their own experiences in introducing the books to their friends and neighbors. Here are just a few excerpts of some of the many letters from Sierra Leone:**

From Ms. S.A., Koidu Town (spring 1991):

> "First of all, thank you for sending the books to me. The book is useful to me and the people I am counseling. I am carrying out counseling to youth clubs, schools, hospitals and to individuals. I am really having a hard time with most people but a few are starting to accept the facts. Unfortunately, excision is a Secret Society practice here in Sierra Leone and the Society [Bundu Society] is part of our tradition and custom. One should not talk about it if one is not a member of the Society. The Chiefs are encouraging excision out of ignorance. When I tell a Chief to stop such an act she will say I am telling their secret and I will be imprisoned for that. Those that I have counseled have agreed to stop this dangerous act and are requesting more books. Attached are the names of those who have accepted to stop the practice. It would be very much appreciated if you send books for those who have accepted to stop it and help. They are ready to carry out this program."

From Blama Group, Blama (May 1991):

> "Thank you for your letter and the **Childbirth Picture Book** you sent me. I have just finished reading the book which helps to put the struggle in perspective . . . I have decided to form a special group called Women's International Network, Blama Group' . . . Although female circumcision is traditional in this country I have started educating my family and some of my friends about it. I very much hope you can help me by sending more books. . ."

From Women Birth & Nutrition Centre, Kono District (June 1991):

"Thank you so much for your wonderful work. . . Your **Childbirth Picture Book** is helping us here greatly. The materials enclosed in the book are helping us in our teaching against female circumcision. Besides I am giving training to traditional birth attendants. We have been successful in winning the hearts of the women who were engaged in female circumcision. Many women have now pledged their loyalty and support to avoid female circumcision. Those who now know the dangers are helping to teach people who are engaged in it. To succeed in educating more participants on female circumcision I am asking you for more picture books. . ."

From Ms. F.S., Kenema (February 1993):

"I wish to apply for 20 copies of the **Universal Childbirth Picture Book**. I am a village health worker in one of the remote villages of Sierra Leone. I took a course for traditional birth attendants (TBAs) and recently got my certificate and was sent to a village to teach women on childbirth. I use advice from the **Universal Childbirth Picture Book**. I teach the people to forget about female circumcision - especially those who bore female children. I would like more books. I am covering over 30 villages on my teaching rounds. I use the books to illustrate why they should change. I hereby promise that my daughters will not be circumcised. . . Hoping that you will send these materials soon. . ."

From A.K.F., Kissytown, Kenema (July 1993):

"I have formed a club called 'Youth Organization Club' in our village of boys and girls. The purpose of this club is to go around the other villages to tell people about the damage of female circumcision . . . We are succeeding a little bit. A few people have started following our advice. Some have started sending their daughters to our city and larger towns since this is the only way to prevent their girls from being circumcised. As chairman of the above-named club, I would appreciate it much if you can please send us some more of your books . . ."

From Ms. E.G., Makeni Town (February 1993):

"I wish to appeal to you for your most educative teaching material - the **Childbirth Picture Book**. I introduce myself as a state registered nurse attached to the government hospital in Makeni. My work in the hospital is to teach families and junior health workers in health care education. Our centre of concentration is on youths respectively women. . . The mobile clinic comprises other health staff from many other health centres. . . The staff will in turn teach other people in their various clinics when they shall have returned to their various health centres. I should therefore ask for 50 copies of the **Childbirth Picture Book** to be distributed among the health workers. . . The 50 copies will serve as teaching materials to educate those in the rural areas not to engage in female circumcision citing the dangers of this practice."

Many letters are sent by men, often health workers or teachers who write to ask for more Childbirth Picture Books. A high school principal in Kenema, a small market center in the eastern province, organized a program and meetings using the **CBPBs**. He mobilized community groups in the area to work with him and organized discussions all over the region. **WIN NEWS** has more requests for books from Sierra Leone than from anywhere else. Some even send photographs of groups of people looking at the pictures of the books. **CBPBs** are also distributed at local markets with young people crowding around, so the photographs show.

Some of the letter writers report that women who make a living from the operations get angry when they see that the books show what they keep secret - the facts about reproduction. They tell families that their daughters need to be initiated to have children and should be sent to the Bundu bush. But the truth about excision is graphically represented in the **Additions on Excision of the Childbirth Picture Books**. These women will have to be trained in other ways to make a living, as the plan of Dr. Koso-Thomas proposes. Among the programs the Inter-African Committee has developed and sponsored are training programs for excisors.

THE GENERATION GAP

The generation gap is evident and growing all over Africa, especially in urban areas. **Grandmothers are highly respected, and their influence is very strong, especially on their granddaughters.** Most of the older generation has no formal education and almost all older women are illiterate. Given the extended family structure they have considerable control over the young wives married to their sons - for instance, in preventing their daughters-in-law from using contraceptives. **Where households are segregated, as in Sudan, the battle between generations of women often decides the future and fate of today's children. This generation gap, repeated all over Africa, will continue until the younger generation reaches maturity,** as this story from Sudan documents:

> "Nour, a 60-year-old grandmother, lives with her family in Khartoum. A member of the Hadendowa tribe, she was circumcised Pharaonic style at the age of 7. The shock and pain of this ritual . . . was repeated for Nour each time she gave birth, hanging traditional style, arms and hands tied to the ceiling. Each time, she suffered the torture of rupturing the tightly sewn area, resewn after each birth according to tradition. Her eldest daughter, Fathia, is now 30 years old. Unlike her mother, she was not infibulated but excised with only the clitoris removed.
>
> Nour and Fathia are engaged in a bitter conflict over Fathia's 7-year-old daughter, Siham. The grandmother believes it is time for her to be operated, like all good Sudanese girls; Fathia is vehemently opposed to the practice. A university graduate who has traveled in Europe, Fathia, like her friends, has begun to rebel against the sufferings caused to women by these old practices. She considers herself lucky to have escaped with only excision, but freely admits the problems she has had as a result, the pain and lack of sexual satisfaction caused by the mutilation. She is determined that her daughter will not suffer the same fate.
>
> The dialogue between Nour and Fathia has become the classic conflict between old and new generation Sudanese women. The men tacitly support the practice. Driven by a fear that unless the child is circumcised she will never be able to attract a husband, grandmothers have been known to defy mothers and solve the argument by secretly taking the children to a traditional midwife.
>
> It is a common belief among the old women - a belief usually encouraged by midwives who make their living from these operations - that unless the introitus is tightened by the operation a girl cannot please a man.
>
> Divorce, according to local tradition supported by the government, is still an easy process in the Sudan. A man can simply throw his wife out and take another. Grandmothers fear divorce and do everything possible to make their granddaughters attractive to men; the midwives claim that the operations will do it."

A survey conducted by Asma Dareer, M.D., which includes thousands of interviews with Sudanese men and women all over the northern provinces, is documented in her 1982 book, **Woman, Why Do You Weep?** It documents that the vast majority of the people, and especially men, firmly support infibulation. Indeed, most men want their wives to be re-infibulated after each birth, making the reproductive life of each woman a continuous torture.

The generation gap is visible all over Africa, especially since many older people, respected for their age, have no formal education. Most older women are illiterate and alienated from all modernization, which they perceive as a threat to their authority bestowed by age. As a result they desperately cling to tradition which guarantees them respect. Grandparents - and especially grandmothers - insist on maintaining all customs including genital mutilation because not to do so would be to admit that their suffering has been in vain.

There are many stories told all over Africa of young parents, living and working in cities, who visit their families in their rural homes during vacations or family gatherings. The grandmothers use these opportunities to lure their granddaughters to the local midwives and have them operated even if they know that the parents are opposed. **They are convinced that the operation is essential for a girl's success in life and will guarantee a good marriage.** The idea that today some educated men may reject women who are mutilated simply does not occur to them.

When I first visited Ouagadougou, Burkina Faso, to show the French translation of the **Childbirth Picture Books** with the **Additions to Prevent Excision and Infibulation** to the Health Ministry, I also talked to the WHO representative and asked how widespread the practice of FGM was. A young man who worked in the WHO office spoke up:

> "I am a Mossi, and all Mossis excise their girls. It is the tradition. But some of my friends and I - we all work for the government - refuse to have our daughters done because we know the problems. The older generation, our parents and the grandparents especially, they insist on it. Some just take the grandchildren and have them operated on behind their parents' backs. It happens all the time. But I have solved this problem in my family. I told my wife that I hold her responsible; if she does not watch out when we visit our parents and something happens to my daughters, I shall divorce her. I don't want to see her or my daughters ever again."

This is one way to solve the problem in this society, where all family decisions and especially decisions about the operations are still made entirely by men. **The generation gap is a problem all over Africa. Nowhere has education reached the older generation,** who have quite literally been left out as far as change is concerned.

Deeply ingrained tradition combined with respect for the older generation can result in tragedy for the next generation, as this story, related by Awa Thiam in her book **La Parole aux Negresses,** shows. It was told to her by a young mother of two daughters who returned to Mali after getting a university degree in France:

> "After I became conscious of all the problems that result from genital operations, my husband and I decided that we would not allow our children to be either excised or infibulated. My children were born in France, where both my husband and I finished our studies. When we returned to Mali, my mother was the first to ask if I had the girls excised and infibulated. I said no and that I was opposed to it.
>
> During their vacations, after I had found a job, I often left my children with my mother during the day and came to fetch them for the weekend. One day, coming home from work, I passed by their house to say hello to the girls but I didn't see them playing outside. So I asked my mother, 'Where are they?' 'Oh, they are in their room,' she said. I went inside. They were lying on the floor on some mats. Their swollen eyes and faces took my breath away, and I screamed: 'What has happened to you?' But before they could answer, my mother replied: **'Don't trouble yourself about my little girls. I had them excised and infibulated this morning.'**
>
> I cannot say what I felt at that moment. What could I do against my mother? I felt revolt rising in me, but I was helpless against her. My first reaction was to cry. She said: 'You should be very happy. Everything went well with the girls.' Rather than being disrespectful, which is very badly taken in our society in Mali, I quickly left. I believe nothing will change unless women begin to organize and openly discuss their objections to these practices and educate their families on why this must stop."

Some little girls hear about the celebrations that make them the center of attention and especially the presents. **Therefore they ask to undergo the ceremony,** not knowing what really takes place. **A young mother tells how she dealt with this:**

> "When my first daughter had reached the age of 6 she began to ask me about initiation. She had heard from her friends in school about the presents and celebrations. 'I want to be like my friends; I want to be excised, she said.' She did not know of course what it meant. She asked again and again, no doubt her grandmother was also involved. I realized I had to do something so I told her I would get everything ready. The next day, when we were alone, I made her sit on a stool and told her to open her legs wide. I asked her to put her hands over her eyes and never to look but to be courageous and not to cry. Then I squeezed her clitoris with my fingers and took a table knife and touched the clitoris so she could feel the cold metal on her warm skin. Finally I said, 'This is it, now you are excised like all the others,' and I gave her a present as is customary so she could show it to her friends.
>
> Now my daughter is 20 and of course she knows she has not been excised. But since she is an adult she can decide for herself what to do."

Many young people leave the rural areas to get an education in the cities as higher education is not available in the villages. Most remain permanently in the towns where they have trained, and try to get work and settle there. The rapid growth of cities and towns all over Africa confirms this movement from rural to urban areas. It started in Africa only about 25 years ago and at present is in full swing. Modernization and urbanization go hand in hand, and few young people return to the rural areas, which have remained in the past. **This tragic story was told by a young schoolteacher from a very traditional rural area in western Mali. After years of training and then teaching in a town he returned to visit his family for the initiation of his youngest sister:**

"I am the second son of my mother. She had 13 children; only three remained - my older brother who lives near my parents, my youngest sister who was still a child when I left, and myself. My sister was a happy girl and loved by everyone in our village; she was special as the youngest daughter of the village chief.

It is our custom that at the age of 18, when the girls want to get married, they have to go through excision. The time came for my sister to be excised. On the appointed day, very early in the morning, my sister, with other village girls, was taken outside the village to the place where these ceremonies are usually conducted. A little while later some of the old women who take care of the operations came to our house and said that there were some complications.

The other girls had come back to the village, accompanied by tam tams. In our society excision is an occasion for a great festival, with no expenses spared by the parents of the girl and the parents of the boy the girl is promised to marry. I came to participate in this special occasion. In the evening, my sister was carried back to our house very ill. We called the medicine man, who tried to stop her bleeding that had developed from the operation. I tried to contact a doctor or hospital, but the nearest one was many hours away and my sister was too weak to travel.

She continued to bleed throughout the night. The news had been passed around in the village, everybody worried as she was the oldest of her group, and her accident ruined the festival. After a night of great pain, she died early the next morning. My mother, who had lost her 11th child and last daughter, collapsed completely and wanted to kill herself. She had to be watched, to keep her from committing suicide. Even today, after many years, she speaks to me about it.

In all the surrounding villages the news of my sister's death spread because my father as village chief was highly respected. Since that event excision, which formerly was an important occasion for people in the whole region to show their wealth and social status, has lost its prestige. Other girls died from excision before my sister, but because of the status of my father, and because my sister was liked so well, her tragic and unnecessary death made the people realize the danger of these operations.

To be sure, excision has not yet vanished from our area, but it has lost the magic of former times. The traditionalists still continue with it . . . I shall never allow my daughters to be excised. I wanted to talk to my parents before my sister was operated but out of respect I did not dare to do so, as I had just returned and was a guest as well as a son. But I shall speak against it now everywhere, because I do not want that others lose their sisters or their daughters whom they love in this terrible way, **like a lovely flower that was destroyed for no reason at all."**

Neither the young teacher who told about the needless death of his sister nor anyone speaking about these damaging traditions ever blames the operators, even where they promote the operations purely on economic grounds. **They are everywhere perceived to perform an important service, and even if a child dies, this is fate or due to evil spirits or even the fault of the girl, but the excisor is never blamed.** To the traditional dangers of the mutilations of uncontrolled bleeding, infections and tetanus, HIV/AIDS infection has been added, especially in group operations where the same cutting tool is used for all. Though no definitive research has been done, it is clear that cuts or skin abrasions in the genital area involving bleeding heighten the possibility of infection. Statistics by WHO show that Africa has the highest HIV/AIDS infection rates in the world.

The generation gap in Kenya, as in other parts of Africa, is enhanced by the gap between urban and rural living conditions. In the village it is impossible to keep secrets, everyone knows his or her neighbors affairs. Urban life offers anonymity but also isolation, yet it is there where not only the seeds of change are planted through education but where new ideas are protected from interference by others who oppose anything new. **A middle-aged Kenyan woman, working in Nairobi, tells how she escaped excision many years ago:**

I am now nearly 50 years old - and when I was a girl I was one of the few to escape from being excised, though all other girls in my village were. Without it you could not get married. At the time the practice was universal in all rural areas of our country except for the Luo who never did it. I was sent to a Protestant missionary school; they did not believe in the operations and protected girls who did not want to do it. Initiation, including excision, was later promoted all over the country by our leader Kenyatta who became our first president; therefore I never dared to talk about this.

With the help of my school I got a job in Nairobi and only went back to my village to visit during the times when excisions did not take place; initiations were organized at certain times of the year usually after the harvest as a lot of feasting and eating was involved. Of course the excised girls were kept outside the village and did not take part in the feast; they had to take care of their wounds and were in great pain. I avoided visiting at that time. Fortunately no one asked me after my mother died.

The people who ran the school helped me, but the pressure to be initiated and excised was enormous. If it was known that you were not, no one would speak to you, and you were rejected and excluded from all social affairs, teased and ridiculed by your peers. Both my sisters were initiated because they could not stand the pressure at that time; it was practically made out to be a patriotic duty.

Most of my friends are excised due to pressure by their families; it was implied that unless a girl was excised she could not be married, she was not an adult nor a respected member of her family and community. I only escaped this ordeal to which all my contemporaries were subjected due to some fortunate circumstances and because I never talked about it to anyone until now. My husband is one of the few men who rejects these damaging customs; he went to the same school as I did and believes that a man who requires a mutilated wife has no self respect.

Now things are changing, and in Nairobi the issue is slowly beginning to be discussed since President Moi spoke against it several times. But girls are still sent to their grandparents in the villages where initiations continue. Among the new generation, that is, the daughters of my children, few are being excised among those who work for the government or are professionals. But in the rural areas little has changed, especially among the believers in tradition, and many still do it."

Finally, an excisor should speak for herself. As stated above, excisors are greatly respected in their communities for performing an important service. In many areas they double as traditional midwives, and everywhere they are greatly rewarded for their work.

Mme. Fatou lives in a small town in the eastern part of Senegal where literally all women are excised. She herself is a Bambara, and Bambara girls now are operated between 3 and 12 years of age.

"I have two women working with me; they hold the girls who come to be operated. I use a sharp knife that I first dip in boiling water. I cut everything between the large lips after taking hold of the skin folds with my nails. Then if the parents ask for this I fix together the two edges of the skin that is left so they stick together permanently and form a scar. But to make it stay closed the girl cannot walk for two weeks; she has to lie still with her legs closed.

Then later when she is married the husband usually comes to see me so that I cut her open. Because he cannot enter her himself, he needs my help. Some men do the cutting themselves, but they don't know where to cut and there are accidents. The husband has to have intercourse often or the opening will close again. I get paid for my services and make a good living, and the parents appreciate my work."

Mme. Yassin lives in a small town in Mali and is an excisor by trade. She is known and respected throughout her community and tells her story:

"I started to work and learn my trade when I was 12 years old. My mother was an excisor from the blacksmith cast, and I learned from her. This is a long time ago when everything was different. We operated on a group of eight to 10 girls often just before they were to get married, when they were 12 to 15 years old. It was forbidden to cry because that dishonors the family. After the excision the girls stayed with us for several weeks, we took care of the wounds with different traditional medicines including ritual baths. There were celebrations held and lessons given on how to behave and show respect to the husband and how to take care of him and the household. The third week after the excision the hair of the girls was cut short.

Now we use alcohol instead of the traditional medicines and razor blades, which we get at the hospital from the midwives who told us about this. In our country the clitoris is regarded as ugly, and it can injure the husband. A woman who is not cut is considered to be disgusting. Therefore the operation is done just before marriage.

It is also said here that the clitoris can kill the baby during the birth or it can prevent conception. Sometimes the parents of the girls come back and demand a second operation if they find that not everything has been cut. The area must be smooth, the clitoris and small lips, all of it has to be removed. I have had hardly any accidents, certainly none in recent years.

Now the parents pay a thousand francs for the operation, and they take the girls home immediately; most of them also are much younger than before. But now the operations are also being done in the hospital right after birth or on young babies. It does not matter much to me; I am known and am making a good living. But my daughter who has started to work with me, from what will she live if the hospital takes over and she can't get any more work?"

In the high-rise apartments of the public housing developments in the suburbs of Paris live many African immigrant families, mostly from Mali, Senegal and other francophone countries. Social workers regularly visit families with children, as required by law, to make sure they are immunized and come to the clinic, especially babies born in France.

When one of the women physicians at the clinic noticed a little African girl of 3 who was cringing, holding her legs together and visibly in pain, she asked the mother. Upon further questioning by the doctor **the Malian woman reluctantly said the child had been excised the week before, and tearfully told her the whole story in broken French:**

"All girls in our families are excised. We can't afford to go home to have it done and the longer you wait the more difficult it is. My husband heard from a friend that a woman excisor from Mali was here and doing the operations for a lot of families. So he engaged her to cut our child. She did it on the kitchen table, she is very strong; she and my husband held the legs of the child; I had to hold her arms. There was a lot of blood at first but fortunately the bleeding stopped after a while. The excisor left right afterwards. I put some alcohol on the wound; she was crying terribly. But now a week later she has calmed down, but when she has to go to the toilet she still cries. We had to do it because it is our custom, and we cannot go home otherwise."

The physician tried to persuade the child to let her examine the wound to see if it was infected, but the little girl would not let the doctor touch her. The doctor gave the mother some antibiotics and asked her to return immediately if she noticed any problems. The husband then came in to fetch them and the doctor tried to talk to him. "This is none of your business," he said, raising his voice, "we can do with our children whatever we want. **You whites have no right to mix in our African customs," and he picked up the child and left, followed three steps behind by his wife.** The young woman physician was stunned.

There had been a number of excision cases in the criminal courts in Paris, but these cases dragged on for years and accomplished nothing for the children involved. As long as France deliberately ignores the situation in Africa, as the French Government has always done, African immigrants in France will continue to practice "their" customs while living in government-subsidized housing, using health services paid for by French taxpayers and going to French schools, while breaking French laws.

A POEM BY DAHABO ELMI MUSE OF SOMALIA

At the international conference on Strategies to Bring About Change, held in Mogadishu, in June 1988, this poem was read by its author at the formal closing session in the Great Hall of the Parliament that was attended by government representatives and diplomatic corps. This international meeting was co-sponsored by SWDO (Somali Women's Democratic Organization) and AIDoS (Italian Association for Women in Development).

The conference was the climax of a joint effort organized by SWDO, the official government-sponsored national women's organization of Somalia which had called on the Italian Government and Italian women to assist in their attempt to stop the damaging tradition of infibulating all female children.

A national conference held six months earlier had reviewed the accomplishments of the more than five-year effort by the women of this country to free their society of these terribly damaging traditions. Among the many initiatives organized to attract the support of all the people was a poetry and song competition. Dramatic presentations and short plays were also created to encourage popular expression and involve as many people as possible to join in the effort to change these customs. The eradication program involved all national institutions, government ministries and educational facilities.

This poem, by Dahabo Elmi Muse, won first prize in the national competition organized by the eradication program:

"Pharaoh, who was cursed by God

Who did not hear the preaching of Moses

Who was led astray from the good word of Torah

Hell was his reward!

Drowning was his fate!

The style of their circumcision,

butchering, bleeding, veins dripping with blood!

Cutting, sewing and tailoring the flesh!

This loathsome act never been cited by Prophet nor

acknowledged by the Hadith!

Non-existing in Abu Hureyra,

No Muslim ever preached it!

Past or present the Koran never preached

it (Pharaonic circumcision)

And if I may think of my wedding night,

awaiting me was caresses, sweet,

kisses, hugging and love.

No, never!

Awaiting me was pain, suffering and sadness

In my wedding bed there I lie groaning,

curling like a wounded animal, victim of feminine pain.

At dawn awaits me ridicule.

My mother announces,

yes she is a virgin.

---

*Female Circumcision - Strategies to Bring About Change - Proceedings of the International Seminar on Female Circumcision, 13-16 June 1988, Mogadishu, Somalia. AIDoS (Italian Association for Women in Development), Via del Giubbonari, 30-6 00186 Rome, Italy.

When fear gets hold of me
When anger seizes my body
When hate becomes my company or companion
I get feminine advice, it is only feminine pain they say,
and feminine pain perishes like all feminine things!
The journey continues, or the struggle continues as modern historians say!
As the good tie of marriage matures
As I submit and sorrow subsides
My belly becomes like a balloon
A glimpse of happiness appears
A hope, a new baby, a new life!
Ah, a new life endangers my life
A baby's birth is death and destruction for me!
It is what my grandmother called the three feminine sorrows
and if may I recall my grandmother said,
the day of circumcision, the wedding night and the birth
of a baby are the three feminine sorrows,
As the birth burst: And I cry for help the battered flesh tears.
No mercy, push they say! It is only feminine pain and feminine pain perishes.
When the spouse decides to break the good tie,
when he concludes divorce and desertion,
I retire with my wounds.
And now hear my appeal!
Appeal for dreams broken
Appeal for my right to live as a whole
Appeal to you and all peace-loving people.
Protect, support, give a hand
to innocent little girls, who do no harm, trusting and
obedient to their parents, elders
and all they know are only smiles.
Initiate them to the world of love not to the world of feminine sorrow!"

WOMEN'S HUMAN RIGHTS AND FEMALE GENITAL MUTILATION

"The mutilation of the genital organs of the female body for any reason whatsoever is a fundamental offense against the human rights of all women in general and specifically against the female children and women who are mutilated."

"THE RIGHT TO HEALTH IS A BASIC HUMAN RIGHT THAT CANNOT BE ABRIDGED."

Many thousands of women and men signed this statement circulated by **Women's International Network NEWS** all over the world starting in 1976. It was addressed to UN Secretary-General Kurt Waldheim and Assistant Secretary Helvi Sipila who had headed the 1975 International Women's Year Conference. The signatures were sent to the Human Rights Office in Geneva attached to a petition duly prepared according to the bureaucratic rules. All of this, including repeated mailings over many years of long lists of signatures from women and men from all over the world, was completely ignored.

I also visited the Human Rights Office in Geneva in 1977 to talk to those in charge, and attended some sessions of the **UN Human Rights Commission** conducted each February/ March to learn where and how women's concerns could be heard. These international human rights debates deal almost exclusively with civil and political rights and the right to free speech. What women consider basic human rights - **the right to food, clothing and shelter, the right to health and personal security, as well as the right to education and gainful employment** - are never discussed at these official meetings. Yet these are the human rights that affect the lives of all people everywhere. The **Human Rights Quarterly,** a comparative international journal published by Johns Hopkins University, invited me to prepare a special issue on women's human rights in connection with the 1980 United Nations Mid-Decade Conference for women, to which women from all over the world contributed. The above definition appears in my introduction. (See below.)

Most international human rights organizations forget that women in many societies are restricted from the public sphere. Political life is the prerogative of men alone, while women are limited to their fathers' or husbands' homes. All over the world women are under-represented wherever political decisions are made, and **in the life and death decisions about peace and war, women traditionally are not heard at all.** A broader and more comprehensive definition of human rights including all people is long overdue.

Human rights - specifically women's human rights - have been discussed in **a special section of WIN NEWS** since 1977. For many years each spring issue has been devoted to an extensive global survey of women's human rights. A review of the **"Country Reports on Human Rights Practices,"** published annually by the Department of State according to Congressional requirement, has been included in **WIN NEWS** for more than 10 years. Due to my extensive lobbying for many years, both with Congress and the Department of State, these Country Reports now contain a section on women for every country covered (193 in the latest report); they also cite female genital mutilation (FGM) in every country where this practice - defined as a human rights violation - persists.

The UN World Conference on Human Rights, held in Vienna, Austria, in June 1993,* for the first time recognized women and women's human rights in an official document, the **Vienna Declaration and Program of Action.** This was largely due to a global campaign that included collecting signatures worldwide by women, who were not ignored this time as the Vienna Declaration shows. Specifically, the UN document **"recognizes the importance of the enjoyment by women of the highest standard of physical and mental health . . ."** and **"a woman's right to accessible and adequate health care."**

In another section of the Declaration, "the World Conference stresses the elimination of all forms of sexual harassment, exploitation and trafficking in women, the elimination of gender bias in the administration of justice and the eradication of any conflicts which may arise between the rights of women and **the harmful effects of certain traditional or customary practices,** cultural prejudices and religious extremism. . ."

*World Conference on Human Rights: Vienna, Austria, June 14-25, 1993; Centre for Human Rights, United Nations, CH-1211 Geneva 10, Switzerland. See **WIN NEWS** Vol. 19, No. 3, Summer 1993, pp. 9-13.

The above statements directly apply to FGM though the term is not used in the document, nor is wife abuse named - rather it is defined as "violence against women."

But it has long been obvious that statements and recommendations, especially if made by an overwhelmingly male-dominated bureaucracy answering to male decision makers and politicians, cannot be relied on; **the real proof is implementation**. The only change since the conference has been the appointment of **a Rapporteur on Violence Against Women** who, as other rapporteurs on different issues, will monitor what is happening in the field and report to the Commission on Human Rights in Geneva.

Certainly **the human rights conference in Vienna achieved international visibility** and some recognition of women's rights, considering that until then women's human rights were entirely ignored. Violations of human rights on gender grounds did not seem worth bothering with, neither to the United Nations - that is, governments - nor to the many nongovernmental organizations all over the world dealing with human rights. All this is continually reported in **WIN NEWS**, in the section on Women and Human Rights.

In 1979, after the World Health Organization (WHO) **seminar on the Traditional Practices Affecting the Health of Women and Children,** where FGM was discussed for the first time in an international governmental meeting, I contacted most international human rights organizations and their publications to persuade them to publish the recommendations of this groundbreaking meeting. **The substance of the recommendations** affects the human rights of African women directly and by implication women's human rights everywhere, as the human rights statement cited above confirms. But all my proposals to human rights organizations were ignored or turned down.

Finally, the editor of **Human Rights Quarterly** offered to publish a special issue on women's human rights for the 1980 UN Mid-Decade Conference. It was my task to find contributors and put it together as guest editor from an international perspective. Under the heading **Symposium: Women and International Human Rights,** this was the first-ever publication on women's human rights and included many important contributions by women leaders. It was published in 1981.

The articles were organized under the headings of "Women's International Human Rights - Instruments and Activities," "The Right to Health and Reproductive Freedom" and "Economic Rights." In the introduction I outlined not only the objective of this publication but a feminist definition of women's human rights not limited to political and civil rights, as the discussions of human rights were then and mostly still are. In the conclusion of the introduction I state:

> "It is a delusion to speak about freedom and human rights as long as there are two worlds, one for women and one for men, **both unequal and both not free** because they are inexorably linked and intertwined. Discrimination against females any-where in the world affects the human rights of all of us everywhere.

> For the first time in history, we are beginning to see a different, cooperative, more caring and peaceful way of life ahead. We are beginning to perceive a new freedom and a new dignity in our personal relationships that are no longer dominated by fear between women and men, but by respect and by mutual understanding of each other's needs. The route to this goal is political, of course. The goal, which is shared by all people, is **freedom for women everywhere in the world**. Men can never hope to achieve their own freedom or human rights unless women, on whom they depend for the creation of life, are free. As long as some of us are not free, none of us are free."

Today, 14 years after this first-ever journal on women's human rights was published, **the international situation where women's human rights are concerned has not substantially changed** - despite the United Nations human rights conference in Vienna. There is much more discussion, many more academic publications, and very little action. Most international human rights organizations, including Amnesty International, ignore wom-en, except as political prisoners. Though wife abuse and violence against women are cited every year as human rights violations by the US Department of State (see above), these widespread international human rights abuses continue to be ignored by all international human rights organizations.

In the special issue on women by the **Human Rights Quarterly** it is pointed out that violations of women's human rights are not only ignored by governments of most countries but also by international law, by international institutions, and by the United Nations. For this reason, the **Convention on the Elimination of All Forms of Discrimination Against Women (CEDAW)** has become the most important human rights document for women and for all people, everywhere in the world.

CEDAW has been ratified by more than 130 countries up to now, though the US still is not one of them. Each country ratifying the document must file an initial report about the condition of women and compliance with the Convention requirements as well as follow-up reports at regular intervals. **IWRAW, the International Women's Rights Action Watch,*** reports on the implementation of CEDAW and all related international human rights activities. IWRAW also has organized conferences coordinated with the annual meetings of the CEDAW committee that hears the country reports. FGM is cited in these reports by some countries, such as Burkina Faso, where the government is involved in initiatives to eradicate the practice.

The right to health is discussed in Article 12 of CEDAW in relation to **access to health services and specifically services related to pregnancy and maternity.** In Article 16 the right **to decide freely and responsibly on the number and spacing of their children** is cited - that is, reproductive rights. FGM, however, denies this right. By subjecting girls to genital mutilations men physically control women's reproduction, inflicting life-long health damage. Yet international human rights organizations have to date ignored FGM to which some **2 million girls all over Africa are annually subjected.** Human rights organizations have done next to nothing to protect women's rights to health anywhere.

Amnesty International was approached by Women's International Network regarding women's human rights and genital mutilation. I repeatedly wrote to their international secretariat in London, asking for their help and cooperation in investigating FGM as they have human rights monitors in most countries. This was turned down as well as all other subsequent requests to speak about FGM as a human rights violation and other violations of women's human rights such as wife abuse. **"This subject is outside our mandate"** was their repeated reply. Indeed, Amnesty International claims that all actions for women's rights are outside their mandate except for women as political prisoners: that is, women persecuted while working for objectives set by and for men or in the service of male political leaders.

The same is true for all human rights organizations, as I established in my repeated inquiries. Finally, in the early 1990's, **Human Rights Watch,** which has offices in New York and Washington as well as contacts all over the world, set up a **Women's Rights Project**** in their Washington office. Since then, the project has published a number of reports on women's human rights violations, for instance, trafficking in Burmese women to Thailand's brothels, the abuse and exploitation of household workers in Kuwait, and "honor crimes" whereby men in Brazil are free to murder their wives.

But this is only one small program of a large international human rights organization that cannot possibly report on the thousands of human rights abuses of women everywhere; they cannot deal with issues such as FGM or the pervasive health rights violations of women in many countries committed under the label of culture and tradition. **And health is a basic human rights issue for women that has been entirely ignored.**

Though more has and is being written and reported on human rights than ever before, consciousness about women's human rights does not seem to have reached many human rights organizations. The agenda is still dominated by large organizations like **Amnesty International which excludes domestic violence and all sex crimes** from their agenda as do all other human rights organizations. According to AI, a man working for them can be cited for his human rights achievements in the political arena; he can then go home, beat and rape his wife, and still be praised by Amnesty International as a "hero."

---

*International Women's Rights Action Watch (IWRAW), Humphrey Institute, 301-19th Ave. South, Minneapolis, MN 55455.

**Human Rights Watch, Women's Rights Project, 1522 K St., N.W., Washington, DC 20005-1202; Dorothy Q. Thomas, contact.

By failing to address the root cause of violence and human rights violations - that is, violence practiced in the family and the private sphere, Amnesty International makes sure that violence in the public sphere will continue to grow. Most other human rights organizations are following Amnesty International's example. It is therefore especially important that the **Country Reports on Human Rights Practices** have broken the silence and are reporting on family violence against women. If we really care about human rights and peace we must stop violence in the family, because it is in the family where children learn to respect human rights.

The deliberate blindness of human rights organizations becomes painfully obvious when it comes to FGM: literally none of them, including large numbers of international organizations, **have ever even cited FGM as a human rights violation.** It is also astonishing to note that in the many years of international human rights actions against segregation or apartheid in South Africa the fact that **seclusion, or purdah - that is, apartheid of women** that continues in Pakistan, parts of India, Bangladesh, Saudi Arabia, Afghanistan, Iran, northern Nigeria and other Moslem areas in Africa, and many other countries and areas - is completely ignored by all human rights organizations. **Segregation of women continues and the human rights of women are systematically violated** with the collusion of governments and all international human rights organizations.

This deliberate exclusion of women's human rights is a blight that affects all national and international human rights initiatives organized by men, though they are, of course, "using" women as volunteers to work for them, and they are using female victims to make their case and gather contributions - which are never used to help women. What is more, most decision-making positions in human rights organizations are held by men.

Why is it not objectionable for a woman to be locked up in her father's or husband's house, her person "secluded" and covered with a black shroud - the few times she is permitted to appear in public - when segregation on racial grounds is universally abhorred? Why is it not regarded a violation of international human rights and publicly condemned for girls and women to be excluded from the public sphere, from education, training and jobs, used as household slaves and to provide sex for the men who "own" them, **when such actions on racial grounds are universally cited as human rights violations?**

The double standard and silence by human rights organizations not only indict them, but encourage male violence against women. Women should withhold all support and contributions until human rights organizations publicly condemn all forms of violence against women - **specifically segregation, seclusion, FGM** and exclusion from public life - and support the implementation of CEDAW as a universal human rights document.

The Country Reports on Human Rights Practices by the Department of State have abandoned the damaging myth that the **abuse of women in the family is a "private matter"** and not a crime because it takes place in the home. Here at last we have a very public document that makes the groundbreaking statement that violence by men against women, their own family members, **is not only a crime but an international one**. The reasoning is that all countries are responsible for protecting their citizens equally - a fact that is stated in most constitutions. But by failing to prosecute men for abusing and often killing their wives and female family members, the governments are committing human rights violations - indeed they are violating their own laws. The US Congress requires the Country Reports to be filed as **they form the basis for international relations**: foreign assistance has to be withdrawn - by law - where human rights violations are documented, unless remedies are instituted by the challenged government.

The Country Reports also set an example in reporting on FGM as a human rights violation: information for these reports is gathered in each country by US embassy staff and private organizations as well as the media. In this way, **the awareness of FGM is increased** as well as other abuses of women, including the very widespread family violence against women that literally goes on everywhere.

Women everywhere are recognizing that we share the same problems and therefore the same objectives. As some women leaders at an international conference recently stated, no matter where we come from and live we share the same goals, only our way of getting there is different. But even the ways of reaching our goals are becoming remarkably similar through effective mutual support. While at the beginning of the UN Decade for Women politically inspired divisions and suspicions separated women from different countries and continents, this has changed. It has become increasingly apparent to women that we all suffer the same problems; discrimination and male violence, especially family violence, know no political boundaries or even cultural barriers. Abuse of women goes on globally, wherever the patriarchal family system prevails; it is a shared problem by women of every culture, color and age.

At both the human rights conference in Vienna in 1993 and the **10th anniversary of the Inter-African Committee (IAC) conference in Addis Ababa** on Traditional Practices Affecting the Health of Women and Children* in April 1994, the shared concerns of women were quite vividly documented.

"Culture" and "tradition" are the key words used by many international human rights organizations, as well as many institutions concerned with development, to ignore - or excuse - violence against women, and especially FGM. Even now, despite the work of the IAC, many claim that **traditions must be protected at any price**. Political leaders everywhere can be heard praising women for "protecting our culture and traditions" - even if cultural practices damage the health of women and children, protect wife abuse and FGM, support the segregation of women and foster ignorance and illiteracy. But all this is now beginning to be challenged.

Berhane Ras-Work, the president of the IAC, expressed this change and new direction most persuasively in her opening speech at the Addis Ababa conference:

> "Ten years ago, at the creation of the Inter-African Committee, the social environment was markedly different in approaching deeply rooted tradition and culture. . . . I am sure that some of **you pioneers still remember the threats you received** because you dared express opposition to female genital mutilation. The subject was taboo and a secret. . . **We in the IAC have taken our responsibility as a commitment** and a challenge. Through education and public mobilization national committees have been able to convince parents of the harmful effects of FGM, early childhood marriage and other damaging practices.

> **At present, these practices are being openly challenged in many African countries:** Religious leaders have disassociated religion from the practice of FGM, doctors and health workers are sending messages on the risks associated with FGM, early marriage and nutritional taboos. Many young mothers and fathers are questioning the validity of the custom, the youth are raising their voices in opposition. There is an awareness taking place **identifying these practices as violence against women.**

> The last few years have brought us a long way in our campaign to end harmful traditional practices. Through hard work and dedication it has been possible to influence decisions and impact a change. **FGM is no more a taboo subject.** And yet, in spite of all the achievements so much remains to be done . . . I call on all of you to work out a common strategy. . ."

And she encouraged all to join forces and support this groundbreaking campaign for girls' and women's human rights and health. Violence against the female majority is no longer protected by secrecy. Women everywhere are speaking up - at last. We must join forces across the world to remove cultural traditional impediments and political boundaries to stop male violence in every form and in every family and society, as Ras-Work stated so well. We can change our societies starting with our own families. We have to first change our own perceptions of who we are: **we have the power to change the world.**

*See conference report in the 1994 Spring and Autumn issues of **WIN NEWS**. Contact: Inter-African Committee (IAC) on Traditional Practices Affecting the Health of Women and Children, 147 rue de Lausanne, CH-1202 Geneva, Switzerland; or c/o ATRCW, P.O. Box 3001, Addis Ababa, Ethiopia; Berhane Ras-Work, president.

Violence, much like all human behavior, is learned in the family where children are socialized by example. As Riane Eisler, the author of **The Chalice and the Blade**, so persuasively shows:

> "Only as we begin to apply one standard to human rights violations, whether they occur inside or outside the family, can we see how the **distinction between the public and private spheres** has served to prevent the application of human rights standards to the most formative and fundamental human relations. . . **For it is through the rule of terror in the family that both women and men learn to accept rule by terror as normal in their own societies or against other groups or nations.** The link between cruelty and violence in the private sphere of the family and the cruelty and violence of scapegoating, authoritarianism, and other forms of oppression and domination in the political sphere is all too real. . ." *

In Somalia, the link between violence in the family and in the public sphere can be conclusively documented. In that society every female child is infibulated by her own family as "tradition" which is enforced by men who require infibulation for marriage which is compulsory. Infibulation, the most fiendishly cruel operation invented by men, is how violence is learned by the boys who see how their sisters are treated. For more than a year, when the US Army was in Somalia, television cameras showed violence routinely perpetrated by boys and young men armed with big guns, laughing and enjoying themselves in destroying all civilized life. **Women and children, victimized by their own families,** were brutalized and starved while well-fed young men, using arms to horde food, seemed totally unconcerned about the suffering they inflicted on their own families.

As Eisler states:

> "Today, as never before in human history, the world stands at a crossroads. On the one side is the well-trodden **path of violence and domination - of man over woman, man over man, parent over child, race over race, nation over nation, and man over nature.** This is the road leading to a world of totalitarian controls and nuclear or ecological disaster. On the other side lies a very different path: the road to a world where our basic civil, political, and economic rights - including protection from domination and violence - will be respected, and our natural environment will be protected from man's fabled 'conquest of nature.' This is the road that could take us to a new era of human partnership and peace. . ." *

The false emphasis on the importance of "culture and tradition" protecting practices that have no place in our world must be finally debunked and abandoned. These practices serve only to brutalize children, teaching them that violence is the way to a successful life.

We talk about "development" and at the same time emphasize the importance of "tradition." **When will it finally be recognized that these two concepts are diametrically opposed and entirely incompatible?** Traditions are designed to support an autocratic patriarchal system of absolute power through violence that opposes not only all change but all democratic institutions, where male elders rule over women who are their slaves.

How can we uphold a hierarchical family structure ruled by a male despot and at the same time preach that this man, whose power is based on ruthless violence in the private sphere, should behave in democratic ways in the public sphere and collaborate with others to achieve economic and political success? He is told his customs and traditions must be preserved to continue the autocratic rule of his family. **As a result of these obvious contradictions, development programs fail** while more than half the population - women and children - are entirely ignored and receive neither education nor modern tools, making a mockery of democracy and development.

Much like violence is learned in the family, so a peaceful way of settling conflicts can be learned. This skill can be translated into negotiating the affairs of state in peaceful ways. Women have a great deal of influence on the socialization of their children, but they are subjected to customs over which they have no control, and their position in each family is rigidly controlled by men - to assure that women serve them, according to custom.

* Guest editorial by Riane Eisler, **WIN NEWS** Vol. 19, No. 4, Autumn 1993, pp. 1-3.

Women are too overburdened with their daily tasks, too isolated and too hemmed in by tradition to be conscious of their own lives, power and abilities. **Only when women are educated, so experience confirms, change begins, and it starts by rejection of customs and traditions that affect women's lives.**

Slowly, change is beginning to take over, and with electronic communication the isolation of women is being broken. **New ideas and influences are reaching women everywhere.** Women are the greatest potential advocates for change, for peace and for the achievement of human rights because of our influence on children. **But women themselves must first be reached,** become convinced that they can change their lives, and then demand recognition of their human rights as well as equality in the market place.

All over the world women are in the forefront, working for peace as the basic foundation of human rights and a productive life. Beginning in the family, women have always functioned as peacemakers and negotiators to achieve viable compromise. Is it not quite counterproductive to exclude women from decision-making positions where their diplomatic skills could benefit whole populations? Most people the world over want nothing so much as peace. The vast majority of women everywhere, from Asian or African villages to Wall Street and in parliaments, agree that peace is the foremost priority for their lives and work. **And women are in the majority everywhere. Why is our message for peace and human rights never heard?** Our record of achieving peaceful cooperation is known and tested through long practice in our families and communities.

As stated many times, health is the most essential need and right of women as the creators and nurturers of children, especially during their early years. Women's knowledge of how their bodies function is essential to have and support a healthy family. **Yet women's rights to control their bodies have been traditionally denied by all patriarchal families and authoritarian countries**: these basic rights are denied by fathers, husbands, male legislators and male religious leadership from the Catholic Church to Moslem sheiks: all of these men build their power on controlling women's bodies and fertility. **Abortion is a prime political issue everywhere in the world:** by prohibiting abortion men control women's bodies, fertility and lives. The same is true of genital mutilation in Africa, which is the traditional way for men to assert their control. The objectives are identical, the means are always violent.

Vital information and health education about reproduction and sexuality are deliberately withheld from young girls and women all over the world in violation of their human rights. It simply is not true that basic health information - how our bodies and our reproductive system function - cannot be globally communicated. The information is deliberately obfuscated and mystified by male moralists, male religious leaders and male medical professionals.

Women and girls suffer the terrible consequences of ignorance. They are subjected to the permanent damage of sexual mutilations to rape and innumerable other damaging practices and infections, including HIV/AIDS, with the knowledge of international development agencies, which run multimillion-dollar development, health and population programs yet claim they "cannot interfere in customs."

After more than 40 years of such activities, and 20 years of multimillion-dollar population programs, the US Agency for International Development has failed to teach women how their own bodies function - denying women their most basic human rights. The huge maternal mortality rate has not been reduced, as recent statistics confirm. I have repeatedly testified in Congress on this subject, but my testimonies have been ignored because development and population programs are enormously profitable especially for all the contractors involved. (See Appendix).

It is a delusion to speak about human rights, and especially about the right to health, while deliberately ignoring the annual sexual mutilation of some 2 million girls all over Africa and a host of other damaging traditional practices due to ignorance about reproduction. In our age of communication **the failure to teach about the biological health facts is inexcusable. It is a crime to mutilate a child no matter what the culture** or mythology used to explain such a violation of human rights.

A child feels pain no matter what her culture or color. The clitoris is the most sensitive part of every woman's body, no matter where she lives, on the Equator or at the North Pole. **It is the ultimate racist claim that because a girl is black or brown she must be subjected to a mutilation because it is her "culture and tradition"** - a mutilation which **would be categorically rejected for a white child.** The time for such justifications for doing nothing is long since past - as Berhane Ras-Work, the president of the IAC, stated. Why then are population and health programs financed by USAID still refusing to take preventive action, despite the fact that the Department of State has repeatedly cited FGM as a human rights violation?*

Information on how our bodies function is a basic human right, because without such understanding it is impossible to exercise our right to health. Reproductive health is the topic of the **Childbirth Picture Book/Program,** which teaches with pictures, as the title states, and can be understood by people everywhere, regardless of language or literacy. This is confirmed by our experience with these self-teaching books in many countries, translated into dozens of languages. The books teach about normal childbirth and reproductive health care and have **Additions to Prevent Excision and Infibulation that graphically show the damage done by FGM to women's bodies** and its terrible effects on childbirth.

The most damaging silence for girls and women is the silence about the essential life-giving biological functions of our bodies, not only in Africa but all over the world. It is a fundamental human rights violation to keep especially girls and women in ignorance about what so vitally affects their well-being and lives, making them prey to vicious sexual abuse and disease. Those who have access to this information have no right to withhold it especially from those most vulnerable - girls and young women. **The silence about reproduction is dictated by old men** in power who run every society - the politicians and military rulers together with religious leaders of every denomination who use their influence to keep women ignorant in order to control and exploit them. In the introduction of all the **Childbirth Picture Books** I state:

> "The failure to learn about the natural biological process of giving life, or how a baby is made, continues to be the cause of great suffering, pain and tragedy, quite needlessly. Yet, millions of women and girls continue to live in fear and ignorance of their own bodies and life-giving functions. In many areas of the world, more women still die of childbirth than of any disease; yet this is entirely and easily preventable. **The biological facts of reproduction continue to be the best-kept secrets in many parts of the world,** often distorted by damaging myths, taboos, and fears that threaten and debase the lives and dignity of women.

> We hope that this book and program will be helpful **by making the vital information on reproductive health accessible and available to women and men, and especially the young, all over the world:** it is designed for those who, so far, have not been reached with this vital information."

The Childbirth Picture Books have proven themselves as excellent teaching tools all over the world during the past 14 years and are especially useful in preventing FGM, as hundreds of letters from community health groups, midwives, teachers, physicians and grass roots organizations confirm. (See Appendix.) The books do not need any experts to introduce them - they are readily understood by everyone.

---

* USAID is an agency of and responsible to the Department of State, Washington DC 20523; J. Brian Atwood, Admnistrator. USAID is financed by taxes - you have a right to demand an accounting from the administrator for their failure to prevent FGM in the programs funded by AID. FGM is a human rights violation cited by the Department of State. In my Congressional testimonies I point out that FGM is being medicalized all over Africa, in part due to the absence of FGM prevention by all USAID-funded programs.

ACTIONS FOR CHANGE: SURVEY OF POSITIVE DEVELOPMENTS

Until 1979, female genital mutilation (FGM) could not be discussed at official international meetings, according to the unwritten code that still prevails among governmental and nongovernmental organizations (NGOs) working internationally in the framework of the United Nations. **Much as wife abuse and violence against women were officially ignored until quite recently,** so-called "cultural practices" including systematic torture, ritual murder and all kinds of mutilations, were excluded from discussion by the UN Human Rights Commission and all other human rights initiatives. The vast majority of these torturous traditional practices have one thing in common: they are inflicted on women and children, mostly female children. Many of these practices permanently damage the health of the victims, sometimes causing their death or resulting in disabilities **that render women subservient and unable to escape male control.**

Human rights organizations, including Amnesty International, to this day deliberately ignore FGM, family abuse of women and girls including rape and incest, and even the murder of women for alleged sexual "misbehavior," for instance, in the Middle East, or wife murder in Brazil and other parts of South America. (See chapter on "Human Rights.")

This code of silence was supported by all international organizations, as I found out when I began to investigate FGM in 1973, after an extended research trip all over Africa where I first heard about FGM. No one was willing to answer any questions or provide any facts. Though I found out that the damage to women's health had been brought to the attention of WHO at an official meeting of African women in the 1960's, WHO refused to take notice and claimed this was not their concern. (See **The HOSKEN REPORT.**)

Two of the organizations I contacted had worked in Africa since colonial times and no doubt had some information: the Anti-Slavery Society and the Minority Rights Group in UK. They repeatedly tried to discourage me from continuing my investigation, claiming that publishing anything on FGM would be terribly damaging on cultural grounds, and refused to provide information. When I did publish what I had learned from visiting African hospitals I was viciously attacked in the British press. It is interesting that after I published **The HOSKEN REPORT**, the Minority Rights Group distributed a small pamphlet summarizing this information. And they published a book on FGM a year after the fourth edition of my report appeared. **But they have never supported any actions in Africa to stop FGM.**

The Catholic Church and many other Christian organizations and missionaries maintain hospitals and health programs all over Africa, and knew all the facts long ago. But with one exception, the Scottish Missionary Church in Kenya, they all participated in the conspiracy of silence about FGM and kept the facts hidden. Since many girls die from the mutilations **these institutions from a legal view share the responsibility for their deaths.**

Until my article on **The Epidemiology of Female Genital Mutilation*** appeared in 1978 in the **Tropical Doctor,** the most widely read international medical journal, WHO, UNICEF and all international NGOs and church groups working in Africa claimed FGM was practiced only in a few remote areas of rural Africa. My carefully documented internationally published research torpedoed this self-serving excuse. But even now, after I have repeatedly published **statistics showing that by now more than 127 million girls and women are mutilated in continental Africa** - and this figure has been steadily increasing with population growth - many international organizations, including all the highly financed population programs, deliberately ignore FGM as well as the health damage done to women and girls.

All the current efforts to eradicate FGM, most of them organized by African women, must be seen in the context of this denial, keeping the victims themselves in ignorance.

Tropical Doctor, Vol. 8 (1978), pp. 150-56. Royal Society of Medicine, 1 Wimpole St., London W1M 8AE, UK.

At present the international development and population contractors of the US Agency for International Development (USAID), who are paid millions for running programs in Africa, continue to pretend FGM is not their concern. **The 1995 population budget of USAID is more than $585 million,** which is taxpayers' money, including from women. But almost nothing is spent by USAID on eradication of FGM. The pretext of "culture and tradition" still continues to be used and promoted by the anthropologists who advise USAID - yet they ignore the African women working to eradicate FGM.

THE WHO SEMINAR IN KHARTOUM ON
TRADITIONAL PRACTICES AFFECTING THE HEALTH OF WOMEN AND CHILDREN

In 1978, when my article in the **Tropical Doctor** for the first time established the fact that FGM was a **major public health problem that affected a huge region of Africa,** WHO had to take notice as medical professionals worldwide learned that WHO had failed for years to address this major public health issue.

Shortly after my article was published I was invited by WHO to participate in the seminar they had started to plan for 1979, to be hosted by Sudan and held in Khartoum. The seminar was organized by the regional office of WHO in Alexandria, Egypt, which was then headed by Dr. Taba. Health ministry representatives from all over Africa were invited to this governmental technical meeting, the first ever to discuss "traditional practices."

Health department delegations from Egypt, Somalia, Djibouti, South Yemen, Oman, Ethiopia, Kenya and Nigeria participated, as well as the host country, Sudan, and an observer from Burkina Faso (then called Upper Volta.) Due to the oil crisis many others from West Africa were unable to come because of transportation problems. **The seminar opened up international discussion on FGM** for the first time.

The Khartoum seminar was, and is, an important milestone: it not only opened discussion about FGM, but all damaging traditions that affect health were on the agenda for action. The hard fought-for recommendations formulated at the seminar provide to this day the most important guidelines for action:

- **Adoption of clear national policies for the abolishment of FGM*;**

- **Establishment of national commissions to coordinate and follow up the activities of the bodies involved including, where appropriate, the enactment of legislation prohibiting the practice;**

- **Intensification of general education of the public, including health education at all levels with special emphasis on the dangers and the undesirability of FGM;**

- **Intensification of education programs for traditional birth attendants, midwives, healers and other practitioners of traditional medicine, to demonstrate the harmful effects of FGM with a view to enlisting their support along with general efforts to abolish this practice.**

The proceedings of the five-day seminar, which included discussions of other damaging practices such as child marriage, food tabus especially during pregnancy, cauterization and more, were **published by the WHO regional office in two volumes** and several languages. No other publication by WHO has ever been in such demand. A chapter of **The HOSKEN REPORT** describes the proceedings in which I participated as a member of the WHO secretariat and where I also presented the opening paper on a global review of FGM.

Arriving at the clear and effective recommendations cited above was a difficult and long, drawn-out fight. Most of the Sudanese physicians of the host delegation as well as the representative of WHO headquarters in Geneva, Dr. Bannerman, a physician from Ghana, insisted that female circumcision, the "mildest" form of FGM, should be allowed as "Africans could not be robbed of their cultural traditions." Dr. Bannerman produced a draft for the recommendations formulated in such an ambiguous way that **they could be interpreted to not only permit the operations but the medicalization of the procedure as well.**

*In 1991 the term "female genital mutilation" (FGM) officially replaced the medically incorrect term "female circumcision," which was used at the time of the seminar.

All the participants at that meeting knew that most traditional circumcisers are illiterate, live all over rural Africa and could never be reached - let alone persuaded - to do this "mildest form" of FGM; only complete prohibition would be effective.

It was the ranking woman physician from Nigeria, Dr. Bertha Johnson, who challenged the proposed wording. As alternate president of the seminar and with support of Dr. T.A. Baasher, the secretary of the seminar from the WHO regional office in Alexandria, Egypt, Dr. Johnson refused to go along with the proposed recommendations.

Every afternoon after the meeting concluded, it was my task to help with the editing of the notes of the morning's discussion. On the afternoon before the last day there still was no agreement on the recommendations, and time was running out. The next morning, **Dr. Baasher introduced a new version that was clear, which recommended complete abolishment and also included training to stop FGM. This was unanimously accepted by all.** The Sudanese physicians who had opposed these changes knew, of course, that recommendations are not binding and that no one would challenge them if they continued to do the operations, which are a source of income for all physicians in Sudan.

WHO headquarters in Geneva has taken credit for the seminar ever since, though they contributed nothing and failed to support implementation of the recommendations.

The importance of the seminar recommendations can be measured by the fact that they are still used, providing guidelines in all African and Middle Eastern countries where FGM continues to be practiced. All international organizations adopted the recommendations including UNICEF, which only reluctantly recognized even the existence of FGM, though UNICEF has failed to support, let alone initiate, any effective actions. The same is true of literally all internationally funded population and health programs, which continue to pretend FGM is not their concern. This demonstrates again what women have charged: population programs are not concerned with women's health but with demographic and political objectives. (See **The HOSKEN REPORT**: "The Politics of FGM.")

THE INTER-AFRICAN COMMITTEE (IAC) ON
TRADITIONAL PRACTICES AFFECTING THE HEALTH OF WOMEN AND CHILDREN

It took from 1979 to 1984 until a follow-up meeting to the Khartoum seminar was held in West Africa, as had been suggested at Khartoum. This seminar, organized by NGOs and African women leaders, was held in Dakar, Senegal, with participation by WHO and UNICEF. **At this meeting the Inter-African Committee (IAC) on "Traditional Practices Affecting the Health of Women and Children" was organized by the African women participants.*** Berhane Ras-Work of Ethiopia was chosen as its president.

The IAC developed an action plan based on the Khartoum recommendations and since then has provided the leadership and the organizational framework for the huge effort to eradicate FGM. By now affiliated groups have been formed in more than 24 African countries with direct IAC support to implement the plan. Three regional conferences have been held since then to review activities and make plans for the coming years. The most recent one, held in April 1994 in Addis Ababa, where the African office of the IAC is located, celebrated the 10th anniversary of the IAC. (See **WIN NEWS,** Spring and Autumn issues, 1994.)

The IAC-affiliated groups in different African countries are NGOs and have support from their respective government ministries as well as from local and international organizations, but they depend almost entirely on international financing. **Burkina Faso is now the only country whose government sponsors a national campaign to eradicate FGM,** ever since the collapse of Somalia, where the Somalian Government had organized a major national initiative with support from Italy.

---

* Seminar on "Traditional Practices Affecting the Health of Women and Children," Dakar, Senegal, Feb. 10-14, 1984. Conference report and recommendations available from Inter-African Committee (IAC), c/o Economic Commission for Africa, ATRCW, P.O. Box 3001, Addis Ababa, Ethiopia; or the IAC, 147 Rue de Lausanne, CH-1202 Geneva, Switzerland. See **WIN NEWS,** Vol. 10, No. 2, Spring 1984, pp. 35-36.

The organization of the IAC has clearly started a new era of action. The false cover of past secrecy of these practices is gone. African women are making their concerns and the issues known. Almost everywhere in Africa FGM is quite openly discussed among women leaders. But it is astonishing that **UNICEF**, which claims to support the eradication of FGM, as well as **WHO** and most of the international organizations working in Africa seem not to have learned from this. They are still stuck in the past, using the same rhetoric about culture and tradition or paying lip service by circulating press releases, or claiming to do "research." But on the grass roots level in Africa, where it counts, there is very little positive action.

UNESCO has always ignored FGM, except for supporting one conference held in Paris nearly 10 years ago. The **United Nations Development Program (UNDP)** claims this is a concern for other UN agencies. The **United Nations Population Fund** (UNFPA) has done more than all other agencies in assisting IAC affiliates in several African countries. UNFPA also gave the 1995 Population Award to Berhane Ras-Work, the IAC president, in a formal ceremony in New York. But the kind of regional effort that is necessary, and that has been successfully carried out to deal with other regional health concerns, is not even talked about at present. (See "Politics of FGM.")

At the 1985 UN Decade Conference for Women in Nairobi, the IAC, which had been organized only a year earlier, **held many meetings and workshops to make their commitment and activities known around the world.** The medical facts were explained by women physicians and reports were presented to overflow audiences by IAC affiliates from many different countries, including **Sudan, Gambia, Nigeria, Sierra Leone, Somalia, Mali, Ghana, Senegal, Togo,** and more. This was a complete change from what had happened at the Mid-Decade Conference in Copenhagen in 1980, where some disgruntled African women, led by Marie Angelique Savane, a journalist from Dakar, loudly protested against any mention of FGM. She gained the attention of the press and was rewarded with a good job by the patriarchal UN establishment in Geneva. As one result, Sweden canceled support for programs to stop FGM as "too controversial."

The success in Nairobi put the IAC firmly on the international agenda. Developing a regional network is an important priority as so many countries are involved. Without such a network each group would compete for scarce funds with all others. What is more, the experience gained by each group is shared with all others. The conferences and regional meetings serve the purpose of exchanging information and support.

The IAC has also developed special training and information campaigns as well as educational and training materials, which are shared, learning from the experience gained by affiliates in different countries. To gain recognition and to make their mission known, the IAC has participated in many conferences in Africa and worldwide. **Berhane Ras-Work has spoken at many international and global meetings, gaining great respect for her important mission** and accomplishments. However, the lack of adequate financial support is a constant problem, since all African countries where FGM is practiced are also desperately poor. When it comes to education, information and health training - the principal activities involved in stopping FGM - continuing financial support is necessary, given the economic situation of most African countries.*

THE INTER-AFRICAN COMMITTEE OF NIGERIA**

The IAC of Nigeria is **headed by Dr. Irene Thomas, the first woman physician** of that country, and the program is coordinated by Elizabeth Alabi, a midwife with both national and international experience. Nigeria is the most populous country of Africa, with many different population groups and customs. However, FGM is practiced by most of the population, and other damaging traditional practices also abound. The IAC in Nigeria has run a series of training and information campaigns, on the federal, state and local level, to sensitize and mobilize communities to work against all harmful traditional practices, involving people from all backgrounds.

---

*For more information on IAC programs and activities, see **The HOSKEN REPORT** chapter on "Women and Health," or write to the IAC. A newsletter and videotape are available.

IAC Nigeria: P.O. Box 6051, Lagos, Nigeria. See **The HOSKEN REPORT: Nigeria.

Many training programs for traditional birth attendants (TBAs) and traditional healers, who are the majority of the health care providers on the grass roots level in Nigeria, have been organized by the Nigerian IAC. In addition, training of trainers programs have been developed: those who complete these programs become members of the IAC. A variety of other training and education programs are continuously carried on to reach the very diverse population of this large country and the many women who are illiterate.

A Plan of Action is developed once a year and a variety of lectures and meetings are designed for different groups of professionals as well as all kinds of organizations. To really effectively work against traditional practices it is necessary to organize comprehensive education and training campaigns to reach all levels of the African populations. The example of Nigeria is important because the country has a leadership position in Africa due to its oil production. **Many of the initiatives and programs are discussed in the IAC newsletter, "Your Task."**

A campaign by the **National Association of Nigerian Nurses and Midwives (NANNM)** was carried out from 1988 to 1990 all over Nigeria. Research preceding the campaign showed that FGM was practiced in 13 of the 19 states, and in five states it is estimated that 90 percent of the women underwent some type of FGM.*

EGYPT: THE CAIRO FAMILY PLANNING ASSOCIATION (CFPA) PROJECT

The first-ever program to stop FGM in Egypt was organized by the Cairo Family Planning Association (CFPA), a private group, several years before the IAC was formed. Aziza Hussein, the director of the Family Planning Association, is a world leader in the population field. Yet none of the other family planning or population programs in Africa have followed her example of taking on the eradication of FGM. **The Egyptian program has the longest experience in initiating a variety of programs and activities** that can set an example in terms of approach and initiatives to reach a variety of groups, especially professionals, in the health care field. Compared with sub-Saharan Africa, Egypt has a very large urban population and a much more developed health and hospital system.

The Egyptian program has also made extensive use of the media, including television, which is watched by a very large part of the population, and it recently affiliated with the IAC. At the 1994 UN population conference in Cairo, world attention was focused on FGM. A meeting on FGM, organized by the CFPA, was held at the NGO Forum of the conference, where Aziza Hussein spoke. As reported by the international press, it was documented that, even now, more than 85 percent of girls in rural Egypt are mutilated. Infibulation is also practiced in the southern part of the country, near the border of Sudan. This after more than 12 years of intensive action and information campaigns by the CFPA, which has much support among health professionals who participate in many programs. (See **The HOSKEN REPORT:** Egypt.)

In their most recent annual report the CFPA states that they succeeded in having information on **the hazards of FGM included in family life education programs and school curricula as well as medical and nurses training programs.** The far-flung activities on many different levels of the CFPA programs certainly set an example. It was, however, a shock when, during the 1994 conference, **CNN showed on worldwide television an excision operation of a 10-year-old girl on a kitchen table in a Cairo apartment,** performed by two men introduced as barbers. It was all done so quickly - evidently the men had had much practice - that the child was unable to even struggle or defend herself. This was shown the day after a CNN interview with President Mubarak of Egypt, who, when asked about FGM, claimed it was not practiced in Egypt.

However, now that the conference is over, instead of passing legislation against the practice, which was announced after the shocking CNN revelations, **the Health Minister has not only proposed to train physicians to do the mutilations, but one leading Islamic authority of Egypt has stated that Islam is not opposed to FGM,** while before the opposite was claimed.

---

*The information on the Nigerian IAC summarized here is documented in detail in **The HOSKEN REPORT** chapters on "Women and Health" and "Case History: Nigeria."

SUDAN: THE NATIONAL COMMITTEE ON TRADITIONAL PRACTICES*

In no other country has FGM been more intensively discussed, researched and written about, or more initiatives and actions organized over many years to stop these practices. **Yet infibulation, the most drastic mutilation, continues throughout northern - or Islamic - Sudan.** Research confirms that the majority of the population supports the practice, with tradition and religion the reasons most often given.

The summary of the extensive investigation, carried out in the early 1980's throughout the northern provinces by Dr. Asma Dareer, who worked in the Ministry of Health, concluded that 87 percent of the men surveyed approved of FGM. The corresponding figure for women was 80 percent.** No other research study on FGM has covered such a large area or provided such in-depth information by questioning family members and tabulating their responses. The study also provides an excellent model of how to organize such research.

After campaigning against FGM since colonial times, using a variety of methods, initiatives and education programs involving the health care system, the schools, the government and community leaders, all of which were strongly supported by the British administration, it was a rude awakening to learn that FGM continued to be not only widely practiced but widely supported. **The study of Dr. Dareer documents that FGM is also widespread in Khartoum and Omdurman,** the twin cities separated by the Nile and the seat of the government of this largest country of Africa.

It was especially disturbing to learn that the vast majority of men, who continue to make all family decisions, approve of having their own daughters mutilated. While in Sudan it is regularly claimed - much as in other countries of Africa - that FGM is a "women's affair," it is men who pay the operators and for the related, often costly celebrations, as women do not control the family budget.

Dr. Dareer's study also confirmed that re-infibulation after childbirth continues to be widely practiced, which is especially damaging as it involves extensive surgery with each birth, despite physicians having claimed a few years earlier that this practice, promoted by traditional birth attendants, was disappearing.

Together with other educated women and men, including physicians, Dr. Dareer organized more initiatives and conferences to eradicate FGM, developing additional recommendations. **The Babiker Badri Scientific Society for Women's Studies, located in Omdurman at the Ahfad College for Women, the first women-only college of Sudan,** held meetings which attracted much attention, and also organized some programs to send some of their women students to teach in nearby villages.

After the Inter-African Committee was formed, a Sudanese affiliate was organized in Khartoum to carry on these activities under the leadership of Dr. Osman Modawi, who for many years had headed the department of obstetrics and gynecology of the University of Khartoum. The present IAC committee, which has developed extensive programs and activities, is an NGO headed by Amna Abdel Rahman Hassan, who has provided strong leadership and participated regularly in IAC regional conferences as an active and leading member.

The work of the IAC in Sudan is backed by years of experience in the field and enjoys the support of the medical faculty and profession, which is very influential in Sudan. But given the very strained economic and political situation that presently exists in Sudan and the Government's strong support of Islamic tradition, any initiatives to radically change the ideas and convictions of this society are, at the very least, difficult.

*Sudan National Committee on Traditional Practices Affecting the Health of Women and Children. Amna Abdel Rahman Hassan, P.O. Box 10418, Khartoum, Sudan. See **WIN NEWS**, Vol. 16, No. 1, Winter 1990.

Woman, Why Do You Weep? Circumcision and Its Consequences, by Dr. Asma El Dareer. London: Zed Press, 1982. See **WIN NEWS**, Vol. 9, No. 2, Spring 1983, pp. 60-61.

***Babiker Badri Scientific Society for Women's Studies,** Ahfad College for Women, P.O. Box 167, Omdurman, Sudan. See also **WIN NEWS**, Vol. 7, No. 4, Autumn 1981, p. 34.

And that is at the heart of the problem, especially in Sudan, where an educated elite including a large group of physicians are well aware of not only the immediate health and medical problems involved with these practices, but also the wider social and economic problems that affect the development of the country. Many physicians in Sudan, and elsewhere, do the mutilations, stating this reduces infections. It is also very lucrative.

The present Sudanese leadership is occupied again with the festering civil war that takes priority over everything else. **But no society can flourish while the health of half the population is seriously compromised and destroyed by clinging to a medieval tradition.**

The valiant efforts, mostly by women, to stop these practices are described in detail in **The HOSKEN REPORT,** which has an extensive chapter on Sudan giving the historic and political background of FGM and describing the many efforts and initiatives to stop these practices over the past 50 years.

The Sudan IAC planned to host the IAC regional meeting in November 1993, but due to political problems it had to be canceled and the conference took place in Addis Ababa in April 1994. However, the Sudan Committee held a successful national conference, so reported the director, Amna Rahman Hassan.

The fact that the WHO seminar in 1979 was hosted by Sudan and held in Khartoum was no accident; it confirms the commitment for change by the professional leadership, especially in health. But as long as the civil war in the South continues, there is little hope that the necessary resources will be devoted to the kind of all-out campaign needed to make a real difference.

BURKINA FASO: THE NATIONAL COMMITTEE AGAINST EXCISION*

Burkina Faso is one of the poorest landlocked countries in Africa. Most of the population lives in the southern part of the country, as **the Sahara in the north is moving steadily southward, covering more and more land every year.** Many men go to neighboring countries, especially Cote d'Ivoire, to earn some money to send to their families, most of whom depend on subsistence farming.

The plight of the women in this very traditional society, most of whom are overburdened with heavy field labor, household chores and continuous childbearing, is infinitely worsened by excision, which is customarily performed just before puberty in often drastic ways. In the rural areas, to not undergo this tradition is practically unheard of, as is pointed out in the remarkable film **"Ma fille ne sera pas excise"** (My Daughter Shall Not Be Excised),** made in Burkina Faso for the campaign to eradicate excision, supported by the Government.

Burkina Faso, which was called Upper Volta until 1983, has undergone some drastic changes and political upheavals that initiated a measure of modernization. But as of the latest count, only 27 percent of the population is literate, which means that some 80 to 90 percent of the women cannot read. A literacy campaign was started six years ago.

Traditionally a woman cannot own land, though her life is spent on growing food for her family. If her husband dies, she is inherited by his family whose male elders decide to whom of the men she will be given. Though this custom has been recently prohibited by the Government, which has passed laws to improve the status of women, especially widows, in the rural areas nothing much has changed. In this agricultural society which depends on subsistence farming, being excluded from property ownership makes women themselves the property of men, who control all resources.

---

*Comite national de lutte contre la pratique de l'excision (CNLPE), B.P. 515/01, Ouagadougou 01, Burkina Faso; Mme. Mariam Lamizana, director.

Film made by Boureima Nikiema in Burkina Faso. To obtain the film, contact the CNLPE (above) or La Mediatheque des Trois Mondes, 63, rue du Cardinal Lemoine, 75005 Paris, France. See also **WIN NEWS, Vol. 16, No. 1, Winter 1990 p. 30.

While in the capital city of Ouagadougou educated women are becoming aware that there are alternatives, that women have rights and can speak for themselves, in rural areas women's lives are disposed of by men whose children they must bear and rear and whose land they are required to farm. The heavy hand of patriarchal tradition does not allow women to even question the status quo let alone work for change or for another way of life they cannot even visualize.

At the Khartoum seminar in 1979, the only observer attending that groundbreaking meeting from francophone Africa was Alice Tiendrebeogo of Burkina Faso, who then headed the national women's organization and until recently was Minister of Basic Education, a pivotal position in a country with a largely illiterate population. In 1988, Tiendrebeogo was one of the main organizers of **a three-day conference on excision in Ouagadougou.** For the first time in a national meeting, with delegates from all over the country and an agenda presented in three local languages besides French, the development of a campaign to abolish FGM was discussed.* The objective was, first of all, to sensitize the people and make families aware that **"excision is bad for women, bad for families, and bad for society."**

The objectives of this remarkable conference are detailed in **The HOSKEN REPORT,** and **WIN NEWS** continuously reports on any new developments. The campaign to abolish FGM is coordinated by Mariam Lamizana who, together with the first lady of the country, Mme. Chantal Compaore, came to Addis Ababa in April 1994 to speak at the IAC conference. Compaore also lent her support to an IAC training seminar held in July 1995, organized by AIDoS (Italian Association of Women in Development) and hosted by the Burkina Faso National Committee. (See **WIN NEWS,** Vol. 21, No. 4, Autumn 1995.)

In Burkina Faso and in much of francophone West Africa, due to very high illiteracy - a legacy of the French colonial administration - and very limited communication in rural areas, **the possibility of a different way of life or new ideas other than what is said to have been decreed by the ancestors, is not accepted** by the patriarchal village leaders. They reject the very notion of change as it inevitably infringes on the power they now enjoy. Moslemization in this traditionally animist society is also growing here as in many other African countries, emphasizing blind faith in Allah, who will take care of everything.

It is for all these reasons that **the film about excision, which was made in a village in Burkina Faso with and by local people, has become an important tool. The people who come to see the movie see themselves and their own concerns reflected on the screen.** The film is used to open up conversation about their own problems among the people in rural areas who have rarely been exposed to movies of any kind. It has become a unique consciousness-raising tool. The campaign has also organized a number of other activities such as training traditional birth attendants as well as community and health workers all over the country. An information center has been organized, also radio and television programs. Radio is able to reach even remote areas and enjoys a large audience.

The campaign has developed a three-year action program and budget, but international financial support from UN agencies such as UNICEF, WHO and UNFPA has been very limited. While in the past the excuse for inaction has always been "but the people and the government do not want change regarding FGM," in Burkina Faso a well-organized campaign is going begging for even limited support. Indeed some scheduled meetings in different parts of the country had to be canceled - so the Committee Report shows - because no funds for transportation were available.

In this very poor country the Government has made a real commitment to eradicate these terribly damaging inherited practices which will continue to prevent the population from improving their own lives. The Netherlands has been the one country that has provided direct support for this important campaign, while the US is shutting down the USAID mission which developed family planning programs. The international community has so far failed to provide the resources and the support needed that could make this campaign against FGM **an example for the rest of Africa.**

---

* National Seminar on Traditional Practices Affecting the Health of Women: The Case of Excision, Proposal for Elimination. May 26-28, 1988. Action Sociale, B.P. 515, Ouagadougou, Burkina Faso. See **WIN NEWS,** Vol. 14, No. 3, Summer 1988, pp. 34-35

KENYA: THE MAENDELEO YA WANAWAKE INITIATIVE*

The Maendeleo Ya Wanawake Organization (MYWO) is the largest and oldest village women's organization of Kenya, dating back to colonial times. Its name literally means "women's progress." MYWO has groups all over the country and therefore has been the target of politicians, most recently KANU, the Government party. However, its previous independence has now been restored.

Under the leadership of Jane Kiano, who was the president of MYWO for many years, an impressive multi-story office building, Maendeleo House, was built at the edge of Uhuru Park, near the University of Nairobi, serving as both the location of the organization's headquarters and as a symbol of women's power.

Maendeleo, which has worked for Kenyan women, especially in rural areas, for many years, **took on in the early 1990's the first-ever comprehensive initiative organized by women to work for the eradication of FGM in Kenya.** But first the present-day facts regarding where and by whom FGM is practiced had to be established, as this information had been deliberately hidden, obfuscated and politicized for many years.

FGM has been a taboo subject in Kenya ever since colonial times. The controversy regarding FGM was politicized and used in the independence campaign against the British, making the mutilation of Kenyan girls a cause celebre, victimizing helpless female children as pawns of both sides.

President-for-life Kenyatta, who led the independence campaign as a young man, distinguished himself with the statement **"No Kikuyu will ever marry a woman who is not circumcised."**** His support of FGM not only resulted in cutting off any discussion about working against these damaging practices, but he is responsible for the needless deaths of thousands of African girls in Kenya and all over Africa, where his opinions were very influential.

Kenyatta claimed that FGM was essential for his people to flourish; anyone who attacked FGM was undermining the social viability of "his" society. But Kenyatta failed to mention that the Luo, the chief political rivals of the Kikuyu in Kenya, practiced neither female nor male circumcision, yet they are and continue to be a large influential ethnic group living in the western part of the country.

Kenyatta charged that the British were out to destroy the Kenyan people by trying to save girls from these damaging mutilations, practiced in many areas of Kenya in most drastic ways. The details of this controversy, which lasted for decades, is documented in **The HOSKEN REPORT - Case Study: Kenya.** It has greatly damaged the movement to eradicate FGM all over Africa and even now is used time and again by traditionalists who still support the practice.

As a result of Kenyatta's influence, which continues to this day, FGM was never discussed by any women's organization since many of the women leaders are Kikuyu. In 1980, at the United Nations Mid-Decade Conference for Women in Copenhagen, the Kenyan women, led by Eddah Gachukia, M.P. (her parliamentary appointment goes back to Kenyatta), refused to talk about FGM claiming no data were available and that it was no longer practiced except in remote areas.

At the 1985 UN Decade Conference for Women in Nairobi, when the Inter-African Committee held a series of discussions on FGM at the NGO Forum, women from all over Africa spoke about the situation in their countries and their plans to eradicate the practice. But not a single Kenyan woman came, let alone spoke.

However, in 1982, three years before the UN conference in Kenya, **President Daniel arap Moi, who was elected after Kenyatta's death, categorically prohibited FGM all over Kenya.** This, after he was told that five girls had died the previous week as a result of excision in a rural area where he had come to visit and speak.

---

* Maendeleo Ya Wanawake Organization, P.O. Box 44412, Nairobi, Kenya; Leah Muuya, project director.

** The Kikuyu are the largest ethnic group of Kenya and have dominated political life.

The prohibition of President Moi extended to all government and missionary hospitals by a formal proclamation released by the Health Ministry. This confirms that FGM was medicalized and performed in hospitals. But this prohibition was not supported by education or actions to enforce it. Therefore it has been generally ignored, even though Moi is reported to have repeated the prohibition several times since 1982.

After so many years of enforced silence it was therefore a remarkable change for Maendeleo to take on the issue. Shortly after the 1991 IAC conference in Addis Ababa, where its delegation learned what women's groups affiliated with the IAC were doing in other countries, Maendeleo began its program with international help.*

Initially research had to be organized because the facts had been deliberately hidden for so many years in order to claim internationally, whenever the subject came up, that the practice was vanishing and/or that no information was available.

The first part of the program was designed to conduct detailed investigations by questionnaires in four different areas of the country where it was known that the local ethnic groups practiced FGM. The basic facts were established about the type of operations, the reasons given, the opinions of the people, as well as who and how many people were involved, their background, education, and more.

The strategy to be developed was to target specific groups with interventions based on their views and the findings of the research. **The research confirmed that not only was FGM very widely practiced, but that many people - both men and women - strongly supported the practice.** The myths surrounding FGM, including that FGM makes childbirth easier, girls are "dirty" unless they are excised, women who are excised are more submissive (assuring the husband's dominance), and FGM prevents promiscuity, are quite similar to those in most of Africa. In addition, the social pressure for a girl is enormous. By tradition she is denied many opportunities such as education and training that are available to her brothers. **Marriage - requiring excision first - is a girl's only option; she is attacked if she does not conform to the rules and she is ostracized and ridiculed by the whole community.** Many young girls leave to go to the nearest town or to Nairobi to escape the mutilation and persecution. But since many are unable to earn a living without any skills or education they often turn to prostitution.

The brideprice for a girl who is operated is higher - hence the incentive for the father to have it done at a young age, before his daughters can protest. And a girl who is excised is considered to be a virgin, which increases her value. Though the research confirms that some women believe in the operations, especially older ones, the data show that many mothers are strongly opposed. Many conflicting opinions are held by the same people, and as in other countries - in Sudan, for instance - it is said FGM is a woman's domain - thus shifting the blame to the female victims whose opinions are generally ignored.

It was, however, established that FGM is decreasing in urban areas and that the less traditional ethnic groups oppose the operations; some even recommended organizing mass information campaigns. This recommendation has been made again and again all over Africa, beginning with the WHO seminar in Khartoum, but nowhere has it been heeded, least of all internationally. Yet international support is essential.

A number of people also recommended that in the future FGM should be done in the hospitals. In fact, the research revealed that the operations are already being done in many local hospitals, though they charge more than the traditional excisors. This goes on, despite the 1982 prohibition by President Moi specifically directed to hospitals.

The medicalization of FGM is rapidly increasing in Africa. To mutilate a child in medically correct ways in government-supported health facilities for a fee is the ultimate perversion of medicine. Yet this is happening not only in Kenya but all over Africa, and no one says anything. WHO has resident representatives and offices in every African country. But these physicians - mostly men - have remained silent.

---

*The program was developed with the technical assistance of the Program for Appropriate Technology in Health (PATH)/Kenya, based in Nairobi, and funded by Population Action International (PAI), an independent, privately funded research organization in Washington, D.C.

But the WHO representatives in Africa have never concerned themselves with FGM. I visited many of them in Africa and discovered they never talked to midwives - who deal with childbearing in all the hospitals and throughout the rural areas - and none of them had even heard of the WHO seminar recommendations made in 1979 in Khartoum which supposedly were communicated by WHO throughout Africa.

Maendeleo, after the research was completed, organized a dissemination workshop in Nairobi hosted by the Program for Appropriate Technology in Health (PATH), which had provided technical advice. A report on this workshop presents a summary of the findings as well as recommendations in three main areas: health care provision, communication, and policy/law. The report also states that the senior deputy director of medical services, Dr. Ochola, who was a guest speaker, admitted that the practice was going on in Kenya's health institutions. Many NGOs working in Kenya also attended the workshop.

This certainly was a considerable departure from the past, when no one would publicly speak on FGM let alone hold a meeting. **Maendeleo is now continuing the project with the help of grants. It will take years to get positive results, requiring a long-term effort and commitment** as this problem has been deliberately ignored for such a long time.

The fact that FGM is now done in hospitals all over the country, as admitted by the Health Ministry representative at the Maendeleo meeting, not only flies in the face of what the profession stands for and what every physician swears to uphold, but it is a violation of human rights and medical ethics. Medicalization was also specifically prohibited by President Moi; WHO headquarters in Geneva opposed it; but a WHO representative of Kenya did not even attend the Maendeleo meeting.

Kenya, a most beautiful country with many natural assets, has lately been beset by many manmade problems and political controversies. **Ethnic and political rivalries are sharpened by the huge population growth, which until recently was the highest in the world** (over 4 percent) and has only marginally been reduced by the multimillion-dollar population programs funded primarily by USAID and the World Bank. **But none of these programs which have trained many people all over Kenya have even looked at FGM - they have deliberately ignored the practice in all project areas** though their people in the field are well aware of the health damage that these practices entail. The many contractors who are funded to carry out population programs deliberately ignore the health of the women - and that must be protested.

Despite all the money spent, rapid population growth in Kenya continues and threatens to overwhelm the country and its resources, heightening ethnic and political rivalries over land - a limited resource. **But as long as every Kenyan man seeks to bolster his ego by fathering more and more children while evading his obligation to support them, which is shifted to women, Kenya's economic problems will only worsen.**

Recently, rape and sexual assaults have been reported more frequently, including the terrible mass sexual assaults and killings at a Catholic boarding school in Meru, where male students overpowered and raped 71 of their female classmates and killed 19 who resisted. This was reported around the world.* **But the Kenyan Government failed to punish the responsible school administrators, one of whom stated: "But the boys did not want to do any harm - they just wanted to rape."**

Many rapes are reported in the local press but not internationally, though HIV/AIDS infections, which are overwhelming Kenya, are spread all over the country by rape and FGM. **The brideprice, polygamy, prostitution, rape and FGM - all these patriarchal practices reinforce male power and violence which in Kenya are heightened by the worsening economic problems,** quite aside from steadily growing ethnic rivalries. The massacres that have taken place in Rwanda and Burundi, both neighbors of Kenya, are based on problems quite similar to those faced by Kenya. But the male leadership of Kenya still fails to examine its own attitudes and customs, which are the principle obstacles to the development of this beautiful country.

---

* See **WIN NEWS**, Vol. 17, No. 4, Autumn 1991, pp. 37-41.

SIERRA LEONE: A COUNTRY-WIDE PLAN TO ERADICATE FGM

Sierra Leone is the only African country where a national plan has been developed to eradicate FGM. Excision is practiced, often in drastic form, by almost the entire population. The eradication plan was developed by Dr. Olayinka Koso-Thomas, who worked for many years for the Health Ministry in Freetown and is presently the regional coordinator for the Inter-African Committee for West Africa.

First, some facts: In Sierra Leone, the secret societies of women, called **Bundu** (sometimes spelled Bondo), still hold much political power. Their counterparts are the secret societies for men, called **Poro. Since these societies organize all social life throughout rural areas they have much political power, traditionally exercised by the influential women chiefs.** Outside influences have recently diminished their power, especially in Freetown. However, only about 15 percent of the population is literate - for women it is much less - and therefore beliefs in traditions, witchcraft and magic are still very strong.

The center part of the secret initiation rites into these women's societies is excision - performed either by the matron in charge of the ceremonies or the "digbas," the traditional excisors. The initiations are conducted in a special area outside each village, the Bundu bush, where no one may enter and from which men are strictly excluded. Since the girls who are initiated, traditionally just before they are married, are sworn to secrecy, it has been difficult to learn the facts of what is involved; however, the health damage to women is not unknown, as women are going in ever larger numbers to the government health clinics wherever they are available.

Each initiate stays in the Bundu bush for several weeks, until her wounds are healed. In cases when a girl dies, it is blamed on evil spirits, or on the girl herself for having done something wrong, or it is said that the ritual was not properly performed; the operator or Bundu matron is never blamed.

The secrecy which surrounds the whole ritual is enhanced by the celebration of marriage of the initiate immediately after she leaves the Bundu bush. She joins the family of the man to whom she has been promised by her father for a brideprice, often becoming a second, third, or fourth wife. (In fact, there is no limit on the number of wives a powerful man may purchase.) The girl is given new clothes and gifts for the occasion to which she greatly looks forward.

The terrible pain of the mutilations is concealed by secrecy. **Women and girls are totally uninformed about the biological functions of their own bodies** and are unaware that the problems women often encounter in childbirth are caused by the operations to which they are subjected at initiation.

The Bundu matrons are among the most highly respected members of each village and community. For the Bundu bush ritual they dress up in colorful costumes with fierce-looking masks and decorations, which are greatly admired and highly prized by Western collectors who generally have no idea these masks serve the purpose to brutally mutilate helpless young girls who sometimes die from this terrible torture. But deaths are never blamed on the matrons though it is known that there is danger involved - which heightens the excitement.

Except for Liberia, the neighboring country where the same or related ethnic groups live, these secret societies and their rituals which have evolved over a long time do not exist anywhere else in Africa. But witchcraft, superstitions of all kinds and beliefs in supernatural magic exist in many different and very damaging forms all over Africa - usually carefully hidden from all outsiders.

In **The HOSKEN REPORT chapter on Sierra Leone, a traditional initiation ceremony is described in detail by an eyewitness who watched the whole performance** in the Bundu bush, including the excision operations. These initiations and mutilations go on to this day all over the country, as health facilities confirm. **Only the Creoles, who live in Freetown and make up less than 2 percent of the population,** refuse to mutilate their children. By not practicing FGM these descendants of repatriated freed slaves are excluded from the secret societies and therefore also excluded from all political power.

Due to the influence of the secret societies, working against FGM in Sierra Leone is especially difficult. For instance, if FGM is discussed at an international meeting in the presence of someone from Sierra Leone, it still frequently happens that she or he will protest and stop all further discussion.

It took great courage for Dr. Koso-Thomas to develop and publish her plan. She received her medical training in the UK and worked for many years in the mother and child health department for the Health Ministry in Freetown, where she had ample opportunity to see first-hand the terrible problems and permanent health damage resulting from FGM. When she decided to pursue a degree in public health at the University of California at Berkeley, after many years of practicing gynecology in Freetown, Dr. Koso-Thomas developed the plan to eradicate FGM throughout Sierra Leone for her thesis. This remarkably comprehensive and detailed program includes an institutional framework accompanied by a budget for 20 years and was later published in book form.*

The objective of the program is the complete elimination of FGM throughout Sierra Leone by dividing up the country into several regions, proceeding in sequence so that the experienced gained can be shared. The plan has two main areas of impact: **Health Education,** to increase knowledge of the dangers of FGM, and **Health Care,** to provide treatment and rehabilitation for the victims of FGM.

Though no accurate statistics are available for the whole country, it is estimated from the data of the Family Planning Clinic in Freetown and from the gynecological experience of Dr. Koso-Thomas **that about 25 to 30 percent of women suffer from urinary fistulae, which result in incontinence, a problem that literally destroys the victims' lives and makes them outcasts from their own families and communities.** There are a host of other debilitating health problems, quite aside from prolonged suffering in childbirth due to obstructed labor, painful menstruation and painful intercourse, often resulting in depression as the women have no way to escape the recurring pain.

Some 87 percent of the girls who undergo FGM require medical treatment, as Dr.Koso-Thomas explains in her book. However, they do not have access to it, especially in rural areas. It is known that about 40 to 45 percent of the women are treated by recognized health facilities, for which the government pays. Therefore the costs to the country of treating a large number of girls after undergoing the mutilations is quite considerable, and it does not stop there. The combined cost of treatment for women in childbirth, which would not be necessary except for excision, and the cost of treating older women **make up a sizable part of the health care budget of the government.**

The strategy developed by Koso-Thomas deals with every aspect of the problem. A **National Committee for the Welfare of Women** is first formed with the collaboration of the Health Ministry, which is in charge of the overall direction of the program, assisted by **provincial councils,** one for each province. In each province a similar strategy will be followed which is staged for successive implementation.

The Health Education plan, which is concerned with eradicating the mutilations, has a special task force, called "fox squads," to deal with the secret societies by infiltrating them with a view to change them from the inside and stopping the mutilations. Positive activities are substituted such as training in health, motherhood, nutrition and child care to reduce the high infant mortality rate, and consciousness-raising about the role of women, information on reproductive health and more.

Sub-groups are formed in each province to work on the grass-roots level, contacting specific sections of the population such as market women, women farmers, women traders, teachers, midwives, health workers, and more. Some groups will visit homes and schools, go to hospitals and meet with community leaders and visit mosques to talk to imams. **That is, an intensive educational effort is planned through personal contact to reach all sections of the population.**

---

*Olayinka Koso-Thomas, M.D., M.P.H., **Circumcision of Women: A Strategy for Eradication.** London: Zed Books, 1987. See also **WIN NEWS,** Vol. 13, No. 3, Summer 1987, pp. 34-35.

These activities require special educational materials, booklets and visuals in keeping with local needs. A special education program is planned for the "digbas," the excisors who do the operations, to teach them other ways to make a living. The officials of the initiation societies will be contacted to persuade them to replace the mutilations with beneficial activities such as education programs for girls about to be married.

Rather than prohibiting or stopping the initiations altogether, which would be very difficult in this very traditional society, the objective is to eliminate the mutilations and to use the initiation proceedings to teach positive skills and provide useful education to cope with the changing educational needs - such as teaching about women's reproductive health, family health, nutrition, and more.

The 20-year budget shows that all the costs involved in financing the program would be amortized after the 20 years by savings achieved in the health care budget, which is constantly increasing due to more and more women seeking assistance in the modern sector for health problems caused by FGM. In the past women went to traditional birth attendants who were unable to help them or worsened their problems.

The Health Care program, the other part of the project, is designed to help the mutilated girls and women. This will of course continue to increase for some time as more and more victims seek help in the modern health care sector rather than the traditional health providers, many of whom promote witchcraft. **By stopping FGM these expenses of caring for mutilated women will gradually decrease and finally stop.**

International assistance is, of course, essential, especially initially, as the author of the program repeatedly states. The budget also includes a list of local contributions in kind, such as office and meeting space; volunteers in all areas; local supplies as needed; contributions from government administrators from different trades; and transportation, vehicles and more, from local people. The plan also proposes that participants will be organized into volunteer teams, sharing a substantial part of the work.

Even from a purely economic view it is clear that such a program could, over time, greatly improve the economic situation of the government through considerable savings in health care, quite aside from the losses in work time due to illness and pain caused by FGM, especially by women working for the government.

Since the late 1980's the economic situation of Sierra Leone has steadily deteriorated - and the same is true in most African countries where FGM is practiced.

Computing the real economic costs of FGM is long overdue. Such statistics that translate FGM into economic costs including hospitalization and treatment, which is paid for by each government, should be prepared by all African and Middle Eastern countries where FGM is practiced. This may be more convincing to governments and international donors than any other form of campaigning for eradication of FGM.

Though some of the proposed initiatives are specifically designed for Sierra Leone, this plan and the budget could be readily adapted for other African countries. In contrast to many other initiatives proposed in other countries, this plan depends on the direct participation of local people on the grass-roots level and their contributions of time and local resources. Therefore the participants have a stake in seeing it succeed. **Dr. Koso-Thomas has made a major contribution by developing this model plan to eradicate FGM.**

In Sierra Leone, more than in any other African country, **the Childbirth Picture Books (CBPBs) with the Additions on Excision have been in great demand and very successful on the grass-roots level,** judging from the many letters **WIN NEWS** continuously receives from local community groups, midwives, health centers and schools from different parts of the country. The requests for more books, especially from people in rural areas and from Kenema (a small town in the center of the country) who wish to teach in their own neighborhoods, is very encouraging. Many people, both women and men, seem to be ready not only to stop these practices in their own families, but despite the power of the secret societies they are going out to show more people the pictures of the damage done by the operations. (See Appendix for excerpts of letters from the recipients of CBPBs.)

PROGRAMS TO ERADICATE FGM: OVERVIEW AND SUMMARY

How very much has changed since the 1979 WHO seminar, which laid the groundwork for the formation of the Inter-African Committee, becomes apparent from what is outlined below. Nearly all African countries that refused in the past to even acknowledge the very existence of FGM are not only talking about these practices as damaging, but are now supporting activities to stop the mutilations.

Besides the countries specifically cited above for their programs and/or plans to stop FGM, several other countries' efforts need to be summarized and their initiatives described.

EAST AFRICA

ETHIOPIA, TANZANIA, UGANDA, ERITREA and **DJIBOUTI** have begun different eradication initiatives. (For a list of addresses, contract the IAC.)

In **ETHIOPIA**, after the most recent political change and the establishment of a new government, a new program to eradicate FGM was organized by the **National Committee on Traditional Practices in Ethiopia (NCTPE)**,* affiliated with the IAC. The IAC also has its African headquarters in Addis Ababa, at the Economic Commission of Africa.

The **NCTPE** action-oriented program was begun last year with support from the Italian Association for Women in Development (AIDoS), which also supported the now defunct program in Somalia and developed extensive educational materials for that purpose. These teaching aids are now being adapted for Ethiopia. FGM is practiced throughout the country: excision in the highlands and in Addis Ababa by the Amhara; infibulation in the areas adjoining Somalia, the Red Sea coast, and by most Moslem groups.

Tradition is still very influential among the poor rural and isolated population, whose misguided observance of these very damaging customs adds to their many problems. Recurrent famines have decimated the population, besides the war for independence by Eritrea which continued until two years ago, when the Mengistu dictatorship was finally defeated. But despite all the hardships many men still insist on mutilating their little daughters in order to get the brideprice - which traditionally is only paid if a girl is excised or infibulated as required by custom and tradition.

In addition, child marriage is very widely practiced even by educated families. In Addis Ababa, during the Mengistu regime, I met a woman administrator for the Ethiopian airline. She came from an influential Ethiopian family, and told me that at age 14, just when she had started high school, her father gave her in marriage to a man more than twice her age who was the Ethiopian ambassador to Greece. She had to run the social life of the embassy while bearing four children in her teens and living in a foreign country with no family to support her.

But many poor girls in rural areas who are married long before they are fully grown often die in childbirth or sustain terrible injuries such as fistulae. The new program of the NCTPE is finally addressing all these problems that damage girls' and women's health and lives, which are an obstacle to development.

In **ERITREA** many of the women who fought in the liberation struggle for years are demanding change; they are working to stop damaging traditions including infibulation, which is practiced throughout the country. An IAC-affiliated group was recently formed to specifically address these problems.

Though only a small part of the population is involved in the practice of FGM in **UGANDA**, an IAC-affiliated committee has been recently organized.

---

*National Committee on Traditional Practices in Ethiopia (NCTPE), P.O. Box 24804, Addis Ababa, Ethiopia. See also **WIN NEWS**, Vol. 21, No. 1, Winter 1995, p. 34.

In **TANZANIA**, FGM is practiced in the northern border areas with Kenya, as FGM is an ethnic practice and the same ethnic groups live in both countries. In 1987, a letter signed "Affected Women" was published in national newspapers - an appeal for help to stop excision. After a study, financed by Norway, established the facts of where excision is practiced and by whom and polled opinions of the people involved, a **"Gender Health Risks" program** was developed, funded by Population Action International. Educational materials and programs were developed locally and workshops for leaders were organized by the Institute for Development Training in North Carolina,* which provided technical assistance.

Many new initiatives and actions were developed to encourage participation in the program, such as all kinds of booklets, printed T-shirts with messages, posters, flip charts and more. A number of local volunteers participated as well as existing national groups who formed a joint plan and sponsored training workshops. The activities were continuously supported by some determined women and the program is now being implemented. This program can provide a good model for other countries and areas.

WEST AFRICA

Besides the groundbreaking programs of the **Nigerian IAC** to prevent FGM, which are probably the most comprehensive in Africa and are run by professionals in the health care field (see above), as well as the government-supported program in **BURKINA FASO** (see above), there are a number of programs in other countries concerned with information and education. Most of them are affiliated with the IAC. The information summarized below is reported in more detail in **The HOSKEN REPORT**.

In **MALI**, where infibulation is also widespread and excision is practiced in quite drastic form, some educational programs to stop FGM were begun several years ago. They were sponsored by the Centre Djoliba in Bamako,** a Catholic education center supported by the Netherlands. The Centre used the French edition of the **Childbirth Picture Books with Additions to Prevent Excision and Infibulation** to teach and distribute to the participants of their programs. Since 1983 **WIN NEWS** also has sent hundreds of the books annually to the midwifery school to give to their students to take along to their work assignments after graduation. The French books have also been sent to the midwifery school in **Burkina Faso** as well as to **COTE D'IVOIRE** and other countries in West Africa (see Appendix for **the WIN NEWS Childbirth Picture Book Campaign**).

The economic situation of **Mali** is steadily deteriorating due to the Structural Adjustment imposed by the World Bank/International Monetary Fund on this and most other West African countries. As a result, all services are now being drastically cut, especially education and health care. Most health services for women are affected, which is clearly visible in the maternities that I have visited over the years. Though the population is still increasing, the maternity services are decreasing and are grossly underfunded, with terrible results for women. Maternal and infant mortality rates in West Africa are the highest in the world due to FGM. They have worsened recently, as UNICEF statistics confirm, due to the austerity and devaluation dictated by the World Bank.

It is difficult to understand how the World Bank/IMF expects these very poor countries to pay debts incurred by governments that no longer exist and in many cases have been repudiated. Women and children often pay for these debts with their lives. It is especially ironic that the World Bank started a "Safe Motherhood" program with an expensive conference in Kenya. This program even now does not acknowledge the existence of FGM, and since it began maternal and infant deaths have greatly increased in Africa, in large part due to World Bank policies. (See **The HOSKEN REPORT**: "Politics of FGM.")

The World Bank policies are shrinking the economies by cutting back government programs and expenditures of West African countries, which as a result are becoming poorer and even less able to repay any debts. In **Mali**, the chief victims were the poorest and most vulnerable sector of the population - women and children - after funding for health services and education was drastically cut.

.*Institute for Development Training, 212 E. Rosemary St., Chapel Hill, NC 27514; Diane Altman, project coordinator. See also **The HOSKEN REPORT**: "Women and Health."

**Centre Djoliba, B.P. 298, Bamako; and AMSOPT, B.P. 653, Bamako, Mali.

At the Gabriel Toure Hospital in Bamako, the largest city hospital of the country, the reasons for the high maternal and infant mortality rates are plain to see. The hospital maternity literally has no medical equipment let alone drugs or medicines; the midwives keep scissors and rubber gloves, their only tools, in their pockets as they are irreplaceable. And as the midwives told me, FGM is now done on babies by a resident excisor right in the hospital, though excision in Mali used to be a puberty rite performed just before marriage. The traditional rituals have been abandoned, but the mutilating surgery continues.

In Mali, where most of the people are illiterate - one of the legacies of the French colonial administration - the population continues to grow rapidly, despite the austerity. Education and health care continue to be drastically cut for lack of funds, forcing women to work even harder to support their families. Meanwhile, more and more, men are turning to religion as a solution: Allah will take care of everything, Allah knows best. Men increasingly can be observed carrying their prayer mats or kneeling by the side of the roads five times a day as prescribed by the Koran.

The situation is very different in **SENEGAL,** where the leading ethnic group that dominates politics and life in Dakar, the Wolofs, do not practice FGM. A recent research study,* however, established that in most of the rest of the country, especially in the eastern region of rural Senegal, FGM - excision and also infibulation in some areas - is practiced and promoted by the Marabouts, the highly respected Moslem leaders. A group affiliated with the IAC has been formed. In 1995 ENDA (Environment and Development in the Third World), under the leadership of Marie Helene Mottin-Sylla, printed a Pulaar translation of the **Childbirth Picture Book** with the **Addition on Excision.**

In the tiny country of **GAMBIA,** where English is the language used by the Government though surrounded on all sides by French-speaking Senegal, FGM is also practiced in often very damaging form. A program was recently organized under the leadership of Safiatou Singateh, the former head of the Gambian Women's Bureau and one of its most effective activists. Singateh established BAFROW, the Foundation for Research on Women's Health, Productivity and the Environment,** which started a series of innovative programs to stop FGM.

In the **GUINEAS, SIERRA LEONE** and **LIBERIA,** along the west coast of Africa, FGM is practiced by most of the population. The program proposal for Sierra Leone is described above.

GUINEA (Conakry) has a very active IAC-affiliated program which was organized by a woman physician. This program enjoys government support and expected to host the IAC conference in 1993, but plans had to be canceled due to a newly elected government. However, the first lady of Guinea came to the 1994 conference in Addis Ababa, where she spoke about the progress the program was making.

In **LIBERIA** FGM is practiced throughout the country by the secret societies, which make any actions against FGM very difficult, much as in Sierra Leone (see above). The country has also been engaged in a continuing civil war for a number of years that must first be settled before any effective eradication initiatives can begin.

In the rest of francophone Africa, that is, **COTE D'IVOIRE, BENIN** and **TOGO,** various educational efforts are being made to stop FGM by different groups, most of them affiliated with the IAC.

In **GHANA,** FGM traditionally was not practiced in Accra and along the coast. But some research studies recently established that in Accra immigrants from northern Ghana now also practice FGM. In the mostly Moslem northern region FGM is very widespread. The **CBPB's** are much appreciated in Ghana, as letters from local groups confirm (see Appendix). An IAC-affiliated program has been active ever since the IAC was formed, and recently legislation was passed prohibiting FGM.

---

*Marie Helene Mottin-Sylla, **Excision in Senegal,** published by **Environment and Development in the Third World (ENDA),** B.P. 3370, Dakar, Senegal.

Foundation for Research on Women's Health, Productivity and the Environment, 214 Tafsir Demba M'bye Road, Tobacco Road Estate, P.O. Box S.K. 2854, Kanifing, Gambia.

In **CHAD**, UNICEF recently sponsored a country-wide survey which showed that FGM is widespread in rural areas and is practiced especially by Roman Catholics. In other African countries such as Kenya and Cote d'Ivoire, FGM is most widely practiced by Catholics with the full knowledge of the Catholic Church and local priests, who are directed by Rome not to interfere. This, ever since a mission from the Pope more than 150 years ago gave official permission to Catholics in Africa to mutilate their female children. This official support of FGM by the church has never been revoked. (See **The HOSKEN REPORT**: "History.")

FGM is widespread in **CENTRAL AFRICA,** which was confirmed in the summer of 1994, when a health survey sponsored by the US Embassy found that about 45 percent of the population practice FGM, more in rural areas. Until then, in the absence of any facts, it was officially claimed that FGM was quite rare - much like what was claimed in the past all over Africa by the international male-dominated leadership including WHO and UNICEF.

In **NIGER**, FGM is mainly practiced in the south by a few population groups. Many more details are reported in **The HOSKEN REPORT**.

At present in most African countries some organized efforts are being made to stop these practices, and most new organizations affiliate with the IAC to benefit from their experience and gain access to their technical support and help with fundraising.

In July 1995 the IAC organized a five-day regional training seminar in Ouagadougou, where representatives from groups working on eradication of FGM in 22 countries participated to learn about communication initiatives and to develop effective campaigns. The seminar was led by Daniela Colombo, president of AIDoS (Italian Association on Women in Development), who had organized the very comprehensive national eradication campaign in Somalia.

This training seminar filled a great need. Much more is needed to support the work of the IAC and their affiliates, but except for UNFPA, other UN agencies have so far failed to provide any effective assistance. Though some northern European countries have recently given some funding, USAID and their multimillion-dollar contractors have utterly failed to even take FGM seriously and have deliberately misled women. (See "Politics of FGM.")

FGM OUTSIDE AFRICA

Immigrants from Africa - as immigrants from all over the world - bring along their customs together with other possessions; it is difficult to persuade anyone to give up what they have always been accustomed to. It seems that, for the sake of their children, immigrants should learn to embrace their new environment and life. The younger generation often pays the bitter price for being looked at as "different" and faces many problems in obtaining education and employment.

There is no doubt that by now all African immigrants know that **FGM is not only unacceptable literally everywhere in the Western world outside Africa and a few Middle Eastern countries, but that it is defined as a punishable criminal offense.** Nevertheless several little African girls in **FRANCE** have died from excision; in one case, a father mutilated his infant daughter using his pocket knife, and the baby died.

In **Paris,** a group of women, most of them African immigrants, organized the Group for the Abolition of Sexual Mutilations (G.A.M.S.),* led by a woman pediatrician, Dr. Marie Helene Franjou, who works at government-funded children's clinics. They initiated a teaching and education program for immigrant women. After the death of three African girls and many court cases, the Government belatedly started in 1993 an information campaign in the Paris suburbs where most African immigrants live. Excision is a criminal offense according to French child abuse laws, and by now a number of cases have been heard in the criminal courts, with mixed results.

*G.A.M.S. (Groupe Femmes pour l'Abolition des Mutilations Sexuelles), 8, cite Prost, 75011 Paris, France. G.A.M.S. was formed in 1983 and became affiliated with the IAC in 1991.

Due to economic problems and unemployment fewer immigrants from Africa come to France, and some Africans, unable to find work, have gone back to Africa. **France, which still has much influence in its former colonies, has ignored FGM in Africa and continues to do so.** No research has been sponsored by France so almost no information on the spread of FGM in francophone Africa has been published. **Even now there is very little factual documentation in Cote d'Ivoire, Mali or Guinea**, while in East Africa and Nigeria a good deal of research and facts have been documented. In the absence of such facts it is much more difficult to develop viable education programs for immigrants.

In 1985, special legislation in BRITAIN was passed after several failed attempts to do so. As a result of the legislation, a program to educate immigrants about the damaging results of FGM was funded by the Government. This program is run by **FORWARD (Foundation for Women's Health Research and Development),*** at the Africa Center in London, directed by Stella Efua Dorkenoo, a Ghanaian woman who has lived in the UK for many years.

A number of education programs for African immigrants have been organized as well as programs to teach British social workers assigned to work in areas where African immigrants live. Fortunately, not a single mutilated child has ever died, while several deaths have been reported in France (see above).

Three years ago **FORWARD organized a conference in London for European organizations concerned about FGM**, to exchange information about teaching programs in which a few North American women also participated. Many educated immigrant women, especially those who have recently arrived in Canada and Europe from Somalia, are now teaching other immigrant families about reproductive health and to stop FGM. **The Childbirth Picture Books**, which were recently translated into Somali, are used by many of these programs, in Canada, Sweden, and the Netherlands.

In most of **EUROPE, where health care is funded by the respective governments,** the health ministries have warned all health facilities about the mutilations. Several cases have been recorded of African immigrants bringing their small girls to public clinics and asking the physicians to excise them. This has also happened in **CANADA**, since Canada has accepted many Somali immigrants. Both the health authorities as well as professional organizations of physicians have warned all concerned that the mutilations, according to Canadian law, are criminal child abuse, and immigrants must be told that these practices are prohibited. Medical societies also have developed information on how to take care of mutilated women especially in childbirth. The Canadian Health Department ordered 2,000 copies of **the Somali Childbirth Picture Book,** which was translated by Somali women in Canada and includes the Addition to Prevent Infibulation.

In **AUSTRALIA, which has recently started to accept many immigrants,** including some from Africa, the issue has also surfaced. Fortunately not a single case of an excision performed in Australia has been medically confirmed, though some of the women immigrants from Africa are mutilated and require special health services.

Although **not a single case of FGM has ever been clinically documented** as having been performed in the **UNITED STATES**, the reason is not that such cases do not exist, but due to the physician/patient privacy requirement and because health care is a private matter in the US rather than a government-funded service, as in Europe or Canada, such information is protected and cannot be made public. But as everywhere else it is certain that immigrants to the US continue their customs. Therefore Congresswoman Patricia Schroeder introduced the **"Federal Prohibition of Female Genital Mutilation Act of 1993,"** which has been updated since and incorporated into the Women's Health Equity Act. The key provision of this legislation is an education and outreach program which makes the Secretary of Health and Human Services responsible for carrying out "appropriate education, preventive and outreach activities in communities that traditionally practice female circumcision, excision and infibulation."

As this book goes to press the legislation still awaits enactment. **WIN NEWS, which has a regular section on FGM** and reported on the above legislation, continues to cover this issue as well as all new developments regarding FGM.

***Foundation for Women's Health Research and Development (FORWARD)**, Africa Center, 38 King St., Covent Garden, London WC2E 8JT, UK.

While in Victorian times some misguided physicians in Britain, driven by greed, tried to use sexual operations as miracle cures to suppress female sexuality, especially among the leading social classes, these operations cannot be compared with the systematic mutilation of all female children as an ethnic requirement. What goes on in Africa affects more than 127 million girls and women and kills thousands annually. What was practiced in 19th-century **Britain** affected a small number of wealthy women whose husbands claimed their wives were "hysterical" and needed to be cured by operations on their genitalia.

At the beginning of this century enterprising physicians in the US tried to introduce these money-making procedures which they learned from their brothers in Britain. Since circumcision of male infants is a very lucrative business, the physicians thought they could persuade mothers to have this done to their daughters as well - thus doubling their income. But women saw through this trick and absolutely refused. In the **chapter on "The Western World" in The HOSKEN REPORT,** additional information is provided on this and all kinds of "cures" proposed by male physicians by cutting up women's genitalia. **But this has nothing at all to do with what is practiced in Africa.**

Finally, in **ASIA,** female circumcision, which is different from what is done in most of Africa (see "Health Facts"), is practiced in **MALAYSIA** and **INDONESIA** by Moslems where it is said to have been imported with Moslemization in the 14th century. It is practiced by no other religious group. Female circumcision was also recently reported among a Moslem sect in Bombay, India. Documentation is given in **The HOSKEN REPORT** and a summary is included in the geographic overview of the chapter on "Women and Health."

Two recent publications contain maps which show that FGM is supposed to be practiced in many other parts of the world. **Neither publication provides any documentation,** current medical or gynecological evidence including case histories, which is the only way to reliably confirm the facts (see Introduction.) It is both misleading and damaging to make such claims without any facts, and it detracts from the important efforts by African women in Africa to eradicate and stop these damaging practices.

Since I have worked on establishing a documented epidemiology since 1973, when nothing had been published, I believe **to spread unfounded rumors that FGM is being practiced all over the world is very damaging** as such publications can be used to say that since these practices are so widespread nothing can be done to stop them.

According to all credible research - that is, documentation based on medical examination - **FGM is an ethnic cultural tradition that originated in Africa and is practiced today among a large part of the population in a vast region of sub-Saharan Africa and some Middle Eastern areas adjoining the African continent.** Similar practices elsewhere in the world have mostly been brought there by immigrants from the above regions, such as in Asia, but are often not accepted by the majority of the local population. Some isolated sexual mutilations - such as on religious grounds - have been recorded in historic texts, which has no significance for the health of the rest of the population. In order to effectively stop FGM it is important to concentrate on the regions where FGM is practiced among the majority of the people causing enormous health damage to the female population.

This is a short summary of what is documented in **The HOSKEN REPORT, published in January 1994, with recent developments added. In WIN NEWS, which I began in 1975, a continuing section on FGM reports new information in every issue. Factual information including names and addresses** is provided with each entry. Once a year a progress report is made of the Grass-roots Campaign to Eradicate FGM using **the Childbirth Picture Books,** which is sponsored by **WIN NEWS.** (See Appendix.) The distribution of the **CBPB's,** reaching people on the community level directly, has been remarkably successful.

In recent years, as documented in hundreds of letters from all different countries in Africa, **change is really beginning to reach many different people.** More and more families are abandoning these damaging traditions - not because they are told to by some foreign program director who comes for a day and gives a talk, but because people who look at the drawings of the books recognize themselves and see the problems that result from the mutilations. Since we all share the same biology we also share the same physical problems where childbirth and reproduction are concerned. **Now it is time to greatly expand this grass-roots initiative to reach more people, and for this we need your support.**

PROGRESS REPORT:
WOMEN'S INTERNATIONAL NETWORK GRASSROOTS CAMPAIGN TO STOP FGM

SEE: WIN NEWS 18-1, WINTER '92, pp. 38-40. WIN NEWS 18-3, SUMMER '92, pp. 30-33.
WIN NEWS 19-4, AUTUMN '93, pp. 29-32. WIN NEWS 20-4, AUTUMN '94, pp. 25-28

THE BACKGROUND AND WHO SEMINAR RECOMMENDATIONS:

The **Childbirth Picture Book (CBPB) Program** was started in 1979 to help implement the Recommendations of the groundbreaking World Health Organization **(WHO) Seminar on Traditional Practices Affecting the Health of Women and Children** where Female Genital Mutilation (FGM) was discussed for the first time at an official meeting.

Government Health Departments from nine African and Middle Eastern countries sent delegations to Sudan which hosted this seminar organized by the WHO Regional Office in Alexandria, Egypt, with participation of the WHO Africa Office in Brazzaville, Congo. **Two of the four Recommendations specifically cite education:**

-   **Intensification of general education of the public, including health education at all levels with special emphasis on the dangers and the undesirability of FGM; and**

-   **Intensification of education programmes for traditional birth attendants, midwives, healers and other practitioners of traditional medicine, to demonstrate the harmful effects of FGM. . .**

The WHO regional office invited me to participate as temporary advisor and member of the Secretariat. My research paper on a global review of FGM introduced the discussion of this subject. The Seminar discussions including all research papers were published a year later in two volumes in several languages and widely distributed. (For copies, write to WHO Publications.)

The Recommendations continue to serve as main guidelines for all preventive activities and programs to eradicate FGM all over Africa. **They were adopted and amplified by the Inter-African Committee (IAC) on Traditional Practices Affecting the Health of Women and Children** which was organized in 1984 at a conference in Dakar to follow-up on the Khartoum Seminar. By now the IAC has affiliates in 24 African countries. (IAC c/o ATRCW, Room 627, P.O. Box 3001, Addis Ababa, Ethiopia, and 147 rue de Lausanne, CH-1202 Geneva, Switzerland).

After the Seminar I tried to find **teaching materials that could be used to implement the Recommendations on health education.** The WHO regional office in Alexandria also invited me half a year after the Seminar to a consultation about implementation of the Recommendations where education and communication were discussed. Though I investigated many international sources including UNICEF, UNESCO, IPPF (International Planned Parenthood Federation) and many other international family planning and family health organizations there was almost nothing available that could be used to **explain the process of reproduction and childbirth in simple, straightforward ways that would be understood regardless of language or literacy, let alone anything to prevent FGM.**

Finally, it became evident that specific educational materials had to be developed for that purpose. Together with a medical artist, Marcia L. Williams, a midwife and other health advisors we developed **the Childbirth Picture Books** and their **Additions to Prevent Excision and Infibulation** page by page over nearly a year. A "prototype" was printed first in loose-leaf form in English and French and this was circulated for nearly two years all over the world to health departments, midwifery schools, physicians and nurses for comments and advice. UNICEF and WHO officers especially in Africa and the Middle East were consulted as well as family planning organizations and childbirth educators everywhere. Their helpful comments and reactions resulted in many improvements. The cross-cultural pictures and format - **teaching with pictures** - was greatly appreciated by reviewers. The persuasive pictures make the message clear by **presenting biologically accurate information** in a straightforward way that readers all over the world can relate to their own bodies.

PRINTING OF CBPBS AND TRANSLATIONS

The first books were printed in 1980/81: **The Basic Childbirth Picture Book,** which is distributed in the US, Canada and the UK and the **Universal Childbirth Picture Book** with **Additions to Prevent Excision and Infibulation.** This was followed by translations into French and Spanish. The Arabic translation was added in 1984 made by request of the population program of the Egyptian Health Ministry who had 10,000 copies printed. The Somali translation was made in 1993 by a group of Somali women in Canada and the Health Ministry of Canada immediately ordered 2,000 copies.

WOMEN'S INTERNATIONAL NETWORK GRASSROOTS CAMPAIGN TO STOP FGM (CONT.)

THE UNIVERSAL CHILDBIRTH PICTURE BOOK PROGRAM (CBPB) TEACHING MATERIALS

- **The Basic CBPB**: English with Text, Short Discussion Guide, Glossary and Resource List.
- **The Universal CBPB**: English/French/Spanish/Arabic/Somali with Text, Discussion Guide, Glossary and Resource List.
- **Addition to Prevent Excision**: English/French/Arabic
- **Addition to Prevent Infibulation**: English/French/Arabic
- **Nutrition Supplement**: English/French/Spanish.

Coordinated with the CBPBs are

- **Flip Charts** (for teachers) 4 x the size of the **CBPB**, with separate Text and Discussion Guide
- **Color Slides** of drawings with Text and Discussion Guide for leaders.

The **Additions**, coordinated with the **Universal CBPB**, were developed at the same time as inserts so the same book can be used all over the world. For African countries **the Excision or Infibulation section** is inserted in the back of the book. **In the Somali translation this insert on infibulation is printed as part of the book** as every Somali woman is infibulated.

TRANSLATIONS, PRINTING AND CBPB DISTRIBUTION AROUND THE WORLD

The books are printed under our copyright in India in nine Indian languages by **CHETNA - Centre for Health Education, Training and Nutrition Awareness** (Lilavatiben Lalbhai's Bunglow Civil Camp Rd., Shahibaug, Ahmedabad-380 004, India). CHETNA, organized by a group of Indian women, is teaching women and developing teaching materials about health and nutrition. The Indian Government ordered 36,000 books in Hindi from CHETNA as soon as they were translated in 1985 and many thousands more have been printed in other Indian languages since then.

In Nepal a translation was made into Nepali by the Center for Women and Development (P.O. Box 8205, Kamaladi, Kathmandu, Nepal) who are printing and distributing the **CBPB**. The **CBPB** has been translated and printed in the **Marshall Islands** and this past year in **Senegal** into Pulaar including the Excision Addition. Recently a translation was made in **Northern Thailand** and other translations are under discussion. **WIN NEWS** invites groups interested in translating and/or distributing the **CBPB** to contact us. Copyright use and technical help are available to qualified nonprofit organizations.

THE CBPB GRASSROOTS COMMUNITY CAMPAIGN TO PREVENT FGM

After the **CBPBs** were printed they were sent to all who had provided comments and help with the prototype. Larger quantities were sent to UNICEF and USAID missions in Africa for distribution to midwifery schools and offers were made to all NGOs with health programs in Africa. On a trip to Africa **in 1984 I introduced the books in English and French to health ministries in 10 countries** affected by FGM and subsequently sent them copies for distribution. In each book a note is included, offering more copies to anyone willing to send an evaluation and information on how the books are used.

In all books sent to areas where FGM is practiced, a message is included asking the recipient to promise that his/her daughters will not be operated and asking the readers to spread the message about the dangers and damage resulting from FGM among their families and community. Additional books are offered to all those sending such a statement. As a result, **WIN NEWS** began to receive requests for more copies from community groups, midwives, teachers, health centers and women's groups all over East and West Africa. **The positive response to this grassroots initiative is very encouraging.** More letters from both women and men promising to stop FGM in their families come every week in English and French; many also describe how they spread the message throughout their communities.

The **CBPBs**, without expensive consultants and international experts or special training programs can be used by almost anyone and are persuasive, as the letters confirm. They are used by maternity clinics and midwives for teaching as well as community health workers, schools, local family planning programs, by many different groups and individuals. **The books can be orally translated and locally adapted as needed** and information can be added, for instance, on local foods.

WOMEN'S INTERNATIONAL NETWORK GRASSROOTS CAMPAIGN TO STOP FGM (CONT.)

CHILDBIRTH THE CAUSE OF 500,000 UNNECESSARY DEATHS

The highest maternal death rates are recorded in countries where FGM is practiced, but WHO has failed to implement the Recommendations of the 1979 Seminar which ask for more training of health workers and especially traditional birth attendants. Though WHO has a **"SAFE MOTHERHOOD PROGRAM" activities under this label have failed to address FGM.** Pregnancy related deaths have recently increased due to the damaging World Bank "adjustment policies" - as UNICEF also reported - forcing African countries to drastically cut all health care and especially **maternity services, which were insufficient even before the cut-backs.**

Visiting hospitals in East and West Africa repeatedly, I have observed the dramatic decline of maternity services. Though WHO and UNICEF have representatives in all African countries they have failed to do anything about the need to improve maternity services. **Maternal mortality rates have increased since the international Safe Motherhood programs started: that means their top-down approach - organizing high level conferences and sponsoring research - is failing to address the real problems** which need to be dealt with on the community level in Africa.(For information contact **WIN NEWS.**)

Rather than paying Washington-based development programs staffed by experts as USAID does, **much more support on the community level is needed** including training, teaching materials, technical help and transportation, as so many who write to **WIN NEWS** for more copies of the **CBPB** have stated and proposed. By funding more local health and maternity services and expanding existing ones many lives could be saved and maternal health improved.

A NEW WAY TO TEACH ABOUT REPRODUCTIVE HEALTH AND PREVENTION OF FGM

A community-based approach is needed to improve the health of childbearing women and to teach about prevention of FGM. Showing the damaging results of FGM - as **the Additions on Excision and Infibulation of theChildbirth Picture Books** do - in secrecy and myths. Therefore the books first explain with pictures and show in graphic form the whole process from conception to birth, demonstrating that **the genital organs of a woman are well made for childbirth and cannot be cut or excised without endangering both mother and baby.**

This message has been accepted in all local communities where the **CBPB** has been distributed, so the thousands of letters **WIN NEWS** has received over the years show. They also show that people in local communities are ready to accept change - indeed eager to work for change and stop damaging traditions. To reinforce this message and improve local health, **training of local women as birth attendants** could be done locally for a few weeks at a time by teams going from area to area. Such a training program that goes to each community - instead of taking the trainees away - could eventually include enough women **to set up local support networks working for health and to stop FGM.**

Another way to improve community health and prevent FGM could be to offer young people who want to go on to higher education scholarships in return for working for two years in rural communities, providing health education, including teaching to prevent FGM.

Scholarships in return for community work in health could also be offered to all who want to study medicine - which would provide them with a practical knowledge what the health needs are in local communities. These scholarships could be financed from abroad for an equal number of women and men. In addition special scholarships could be provided to **train local women in midwifery** who will receive special instructions to teach prevention of FGM.

To isolate FGM prevention programs, which are often designed by outsiders or introduce them as a separate activity, as often happens now, makes it very difficult to reach all community people. **FGM prevention needs to be integrated in existing programs and community based.** Most rural women are overworked and have very little time to come to special meetings as they have to take care of children. Therefore the objective is to make prevention of FGM part of all kinds of activities. The **CBPBs also have the advantage that they can be easily taken home and looked at in privacy** - which many women prefer - and they can be shared with friends and discussed.

These are some ways to prevent FGM and involve communities in health education on the local level; no doubt others can be planned. The objective is to get local people involved to develop their own initiatives to change their communities which cannot be done from outside. **Local IAC affiliates who are now active in many African countries should be consulted and invited to collaborate.**

WOMEN'S INTERNATIONAL NETWORK GRASSROOTS CAMPAIGN TO STOP FGM (CONT.)

TEN YEARS OF EXPERIENCE WITH THE CHILDBIRTH PICTURE BOOKS
For more than 10 years **WIN NEWS has sent the CBPBs to community groups in Africa** in areas where FGM is practiced, as well as to all in other regions interested in using them. The requests have steadily grown. Free books are offered to locally based groups and people in developing countries.

The CBPBs have also been used extensively for teaching by many internationally funded programs all over the world. They can be readily adapted for any ongoing health and family planning programs anywhere in the world. **UNICEF, WHO, UNFPA, US AID and many other governmental as well as NGOs have used the CBPBs by the thousands**. But that is a drop in the bucket compared to the great need for basic information on reproductive health and the damaging misinformation that continues to circulate in many societies. **Sponsorships are greatly needed to distribute many more books locally.**

TRANSLATION AND PRINTING: Our experience and advice are readily available to anyone who wants to translate and or adapt the **CBPBs**. They have to be printed under our copyright in order to prevent commercial exploitation. Permission is provided free to any organization or group interested in translating and printing the **CBPBs** and technical help with adaption is available.

CBPB DISTRIBUTION and TESTING PROPOSAL: Based on 10 years of experience **WIN NEWS** is ready to start **distribution of the CBPBs on a much larger scale** as well as testing the books in selected communities. It is proposed to select two different areas in at least two countries where FGM is practiced. In each case local people shall be involved in the distribution and teaching, as well as in testing the **CBPBs**. **Tests of "before and after"** in form of questionnaires given orally by community health workers are designed to measure **the usefulness of the CBPBs in stopping FGM** and to test if the message of the **CBPB** is understood by those who are given copies of the book. Both readers and non-readers will be included as well as women and men. The budget includes the distribution of at least 3,000 copies in English and French in two different countries in East and West Africa.

In addition to testing the message to stop FGM, the usefulness of the CBPB in teaching basic facts about childbirth and nutrition should also be tested. Changes can be readily made in the pictures or text if needed, as well as adaptions for specific countries or ethnic groups. Based on these results much wider distribution of the **CBPB** should be started in many more areas where FGM continues. .

As the letters cited below show - WIN NEWS receives more every week - the writers express quite frankly their own opinions and ideas how to stop FGM. Once or twice a year since 1985 **WIN NEWS** has printed excerpts of letters received from **CBPB** users. Some letter writers also report reactions from their communities including excisors, some of whom are now joining the campaigns against FGM. **However the majority of the CBPB users in Africa are illiterate and cannot write** which has to be remembered when reading these letters which are mostly from women and men who teach with the **CBPBs** and are leaders in their own communities. Many of the letters **WIN NEWS** receives describe this teaching experience. All praise the approach of teaching with pictures as most effective.

In the INTRODUCTION of the CBPB the objectives are outlined which apply whether the **CBPB** is used in Africa with the Additions for the prevention of FGM or around the world:

> "The failure to learn about the natural biological process of giving life, or how a baby is made, continues to be the cause of great suffering, pain and tragedy; quite needlessly. Yet, millions of women and girls continue to live in fear and ignorance of their own bodies and life-giving functions. . . It is especially important that men begin to see the process of conception and birth from a woman's view, to understand how a child is created and what a woman goes through to give life. . .

> To fulfill his responsibility in the creation of a healthy and happy family, each man needs to know about childbirth and to understand this experience from a woman's view. . . The first need for women and men is to understand the marvelous process of nature that shapes the female body, so we can conceive and nurture a child. . .

> The biological facts of reproduction continue to be the best kept secrets in many parts of the world, often distorted by damaging myths, tabus, and fears that threaten and debase the lives and dignity of women. We hope that this book and program will be helpful by making the vital information on reproductive health accessible and available to women and men, and especially the young, all over the world: it is designed for those who, so far, have not been reached with this vital information."

WOMEN'S INTERNATIONAL NETWORK GRASSROOTS CAMPAIGN TO STOP FGM (CONT.)

LETTERS FROM USERS OF THE CHILDBIRTH PICTURE BOOKS (Excerpts):

From Maternal & Child Health Center, Cross River State, Nigeria (Jan. '95)

- "I wish to express my sincere gratitude to this organisation for their contribution towards safe delivery and prevention of foetal deaths during delivery. I have used this book for the past three years and it has proved to be of immense benefit to the Boki people, Cross River State, in particular and the country as a whole. It is useful both in local communities and urban centres. . . . The book has discouraged people from circumcising their female children, prevent maternal deaths, prevent neonatal deaths and help family planning in the country. . . I wish to request that your organisation kindly send me more copies of the **Childbirth Picture Books** to be used in 10 health districts for teaching and demonstration to pregnant mothers and women of childbearing age. . . We live in the tropical forest where there is a lot of malaria infestation. We drink water from shallow moving streams, wells and rivers. . . I shall continue to communicate with you."

From Ms. C.I.W., Gboko, Nigeria (Jan. '95)

- "We the undersigned, do hereby promise that our daughters will not be circumcised and we shall teach others about the dangers of female circumcision: We shall ask them to join us to stop circumcising all girls in our families and the families of friends. (names and signatures of 50 people follow). This is to bring you knowledge that the **Childbirth Picture Book** is wonderfully useful to me as a Family Planning Counsellor. The illustrations are self-explanatory. You can't do without it. When I started using the book my clients were a bit shy to look at the drawings but now they are used to it. . . I work with women and young people and they enjoy my lectures very much when I am using the book. As a matter of fact I need about fifty (50) more books. Thank you."

From Mr. H.B.T., Segbwema, Sierra Leone (Jan. '95)

- "I am now a student Nurse at the Nixon Memorial Methodist Hospital, Segbwema and deemed it necessary to organize another group. The group is now numbered up to 35 people who had willingly signed that 'they will never allow any of their daughters and the daughters of friends and relations to be circumcised (initiated) which is a traditional act. As there are more interested members, I therefore ask that you send more **Childbirth Picture Books** to be distributed among members. . ."

From Mr. H.S.Y., Freetown, Sierra Leone (Jan. '95)

- "My purpose of writing you this letter is to inform you about the female circumcision in Sierra Leone. The circumcision is widely practiced among the traditional people of the provinces. . . Our African women have a real problem through this circumcision because this operation is done on them at the age of 6 - 15 years. . . I have not been communicating with you because of the terrible war in our country. When I was in the eastern region, I was teaching my people to stop this practice immediately. But since the rebel attack on our township, I lost your address. When you reply, I will show you how the Bondo Society performs the operation, and show you which instrument they use. And again I want you to send books so that I am able to teach my people to stop this unlawful act."

From Ms. C. O., Imani Women's Group, Kenya (Jan. '95)

- "I am very happy to write to you this letter on behalf of the project, to ask you kindly to send us a book entitled **Childbirth Picture Book**. We read one of your copies from our friend of Nanyeri Women's Group and it was very interesting and useful to us. It teaches us more about female changes from childhood to adulthood and many other things. . . We are using it to teach other people. We would like many copies. Yes, the families of the women/men we teach understand the drawings. . . So we shall be very grateful if kindly you will send us the books. . ."

From Mr. S.M.C., Kenema, Sierra Leone (Mar. '95)

- "I am the organiser of the Shero's women's club, and we have just held our 3rd annual meeting at the Kenema town hall which over three thousand women attended from all parts of the eastern region. . . After much discussion on the topic of female circumcision many women asked and after explicitly given the answers many women from different age groups greatly regretted that they were excised. At the end of the meeting every one of them promised not to have their daughters excised as they said there is much suffering during the genital operation. The meeting lasted for about 4 hours and every region representative was given a message together with copies of the **Childbirth Picture Books** so that they will take it as a sample and not only hear about it but also see the pictures. . . Please send more books."

WOMEN'S INTERNATIONAL NETWORK GRASSROOTS CAMPAIGN TO STOP FGM (CONT.)

LETTERS FROM USERS OF THE CHILDBIRTH PICTURE BOOKS (Excerpts): (continued)

From Mr. J.B., Library, Bori-Ogoni, Nigeria (Apr. '95)

- "Thank you for sending twelve **Universal Childbirth Picture Books**. . . The copies have been distributed to interested persons and many more who could not have a copy are asking for it. You may wish to send more copies. They number about twenty (20) persons. . . many of them are living in remote areas. . . Though the library is still scanty, it is serving an important purpose as many health workers within this locality are making use of it, free of charge. To build the library, I have obtained health books and literature from too few health organisations. . ."

From People Against Female Genital Mutilation, Kissidou, Guinea (May '95)

- "I am writing this letter on behalf of the above mentioned organisation to ask you for help in order to improve our activity here in Guinea. . . This organization was founded Sept. 1, 1989 in Gbamga, Liberia. . . to totally discourage the practice of female circumcision and explain to people the danger of mutilating girl children and also bring health awareness. The below are listed reasons: the practice is wicked and violates the right of every girl child to develop physically in a healthy and normal way; it is torture and sexual abuse to remove the sexual organs of the girls and can lead to severe problems with menstruation, intercourse and childbirth, also psychological disturbances even death. . . It is often accompanied by life-long excruciating agony. . . During intercourse the male can't sexually enjoy the female because some of the sexual organs of the female have been removed.

We were really gaining support in Liberia. Because many of the "Zoes" the elderly women who mutilate the girls realized the danger and some desist from doing this. In fact, 25 of these traditional women joined our organization. But because of the war, we were not able to cover the whole of Liberia. When the war drove us from Liberia we moved to the republic of Sierra Leone and tried to establish there. But it was not possible because the area was another war center. When we crossed here to Guinea we realized that the practice was too rampant. In August 1991, we reorganized ourselves and people are listening to our message. But because of the health situation in the refugee camps we have included what we call a Health Club in order to educate the women in the following areas: maternity care // family planning // midwifery and nursing // sexually transmitted diseases // oral rehydration therapy and more. We are asking you to please help us to help our young West African women; we are waiting to hear from you."

From Ms. J.K., Women's Club, Kenema, Sierra Leone (Apr. '95)

- "Application for more Childbirth Picture Books: I am very glad in writing you to tell you that all the materials that you sent were received. . . They were not enough for the large numbers of women. I write with the hope that I too may be sent materials for my own women as I am every day getting new converts who have promised to talk to friends and families not to do such an inhuman practice. . . I am talking to families living in distant places about the dangers of the circumcision of females young or old. . . Would you please send me the requested materials."

From Ms. A.N., Wenchi Brong Ahafo, Ghana, West Africa (Jan. '95)

- "I am very glad that you have sent the **Childbirth Picture Book** to me. You said that I should teach boys and girls about the dangers of female circumcision. I will teach them. . . Teenage pregnancies are more likely to result in prolonged labour which increases the dangers for the mothers and the children. . . I will make sure that all the girls and boys are taking part in learning about this problem. I hereby promise that my daughters will not be circumcised and I shall teach others about the dangers of female circumcision. I shall ask them to join me to stop circumcising all girls in our families and the families of friends. I am looking forward to hearing from you soon. . . . Please send me 14 more books that I shall give to those I will teach. . ."

From Aigbogun Clinic & Maternity, Abudu, Nigeria (Feb. '94)

- "The usefulness of the book is that it talks about human life, and also teaches how to keep us away from trouble in pregnancy. . .Women, families, youth understand the drawings with my explanation and analysis. . . Since you sent me this text book there is a great change in my working place. . . Pregnant women eat what they are supposed to, as a result many of them changed. When I speak about circumcision of females all of them weep. . . some of them now believe that because they are victims of circumcision they bleed seriously during labour. . . They promised not to circumcise their daughters. . . Out of 105 women five are not circumcised."

WOMEN'S INTERNATIONAL NETWORK GRASSROOTS CAMPAIGN TO STOP FGM (CONT.)

LETTERS FROM USERS OF THE CHILDBIRTH PICTURE BOOKS (Excerpts): (continued)

From Ms. E.E., Kissy Mess Mess, Freetown, Sierra Leone (Jan. '95)

- "I thank you a million for the 6 books. My group and I send you our best wishes. . . The books have educated me and other people greatly and taught me about my self. I received the books you sent for us and I was happy about the kindness you do for me. . . I have made a lot of people join us in the hospital and school. . . because I love teaching . . . The book is just like the delivery from the power of darkness, these books have brought us to light. We use these books every blessed day, because people have come to me and they like my lecture. We are appealing to you so that you will send some more books for us. . . We want more **Childbirth Picture Books** and Flip Charts."

From Mr. A.D.K.D., Anloga, Volta Region, Ghana, (Feb. '95)

- "I would like to ask you for a **Childbirth Picture Book** to study from it because in our community, female circumcision is practised by the people especially my family. So I would like you to send one of the **Childbirth Picture Books** to them; it is a bad habit and a stop should be put to it. When I receive this book, I will illustrate directly to them that it must not be done. I am sure if I receive this book I would liberate them from the habit. . . Moreover, I am studying general science and life skills which deal with pregnancy. I believe this book will give more explanation about it."

From Ms. K.A., Nursing School, Parakou, Benin (Apr. '95) - translated

- "The teacher in obstetrics showed the pictures of the **Childbirth Picture Book** during her course and I would very much like to have a copy. It would greatly help my education. Though I have taken a course in nursing I also have to work in obstetrics and therefore I need the book including the part on prevention of excision. I have studied the book and I hope you will send copies."

From Ms. E.E., Agon, Daukwa, Ghana, West Africa (Feb. '95)

- "I am very greatful to tell you about the usefulness of this book. It is a very important book to me and everybody I discussed it with. Every one enjoyed the reading of the book especially women. I am using it to let others around me know who are ignorant about pregnancy. . . On every Friday after we close school, we sit together at some places to talk about how a child is born and look at the drawings. . . Some people have asked me to give your address to them so that they can also write to you. . ."

From Ms. L.N.D., N'Djamena, Chad (Dec. '94) - translated

- "I have received your book and I want to cooperate with your organization to completely eradicate circumcision and other forms of damaging practices. I want to inform you that excision is practiced in all three regions of Chad as initiation ceremony. I want to affirm my participation in the battle of Women's International Network and I join the declaration that my daughters will not be circumcised. Please send me more books."

From Ms. T.F., Abidjan, Cote d'Ivoire (Apr. '94) - translated

- "I thank you so very much for sending us the **Childbirth Picture Book**. I am a social assistant and educator in a Social Planning Centre. I use the book to teach my clients and especially adolescents about their bodies; it is very useful because it enables the students to understand the process of impregnantion and therefore also contraception. I hope you can send more books. 70% of the people I teach cannot read or write, therefore, the pictures are important as they speak for themselves. Thank you for your understanding."

From Ms. F.K., Medical Training Center, Nakuru, Kenya (Feb. '94)

- "I was able to read and use a copy of your book and found it very helpful. . . I am a Registered Nurse, Midwife, Community Health Nurse and I also hold a Diploma in Advanced Nursing. We are involved in training Community Nurses. They do general nursing, midwifery. . . Of course I cannot let them circumcise my daughters under any circumstances. I am teaching my students to go out into the community and to discourage it, having learnt and seen the dangers. . ."

From Mr. H.T., Badou, Togo (May '95) - translated

- "Request for **Childbirth Picture Books**: We greatly desire and respectfully request more books to better study about reproduction and birth. I have already contacted about 40 women to form a study group, but they will learn much better with books which we need."

ABOUT THE AUTHOR

Fran P. Hosken is the editor and publisher of **Women's International Network NEWS** - an "open participatory worldwide quarterly journal by, for and about women" - which she started in 1975 to report news on women and development from all over the world. A section on Female Genital Mutilation is included in every issue. **WIN NEWS also** publishes **The HOSKEN REPORT - Genital and Sexual Mutilation of Females** (fourth edition 1994) and **The Childbirth Picture Book/Program** with Additions to Prevent Excision and Infibulation, in several languages, with pictures by Marcia Williams.

An architect and urban planner by profession, she received a master's degree from the Harvard Graduate School of Design and studied city planning at the Massachusetts Institute of Technology. She has worked as a journalist for many years, publishing on architecture, housing, international urban development and women's issues all over the world, and was correspondent-at-large for the **Architectural Forum.** Her books include **The Kathmandu Valley Towns** (Weatherhill), **The Language of Cities** (MacMillan) and **The Functions of Cities** (Schenkman), and she is the author of many professional reports on housing and urban development.

Fran P. Hosken speaks, reads and writes several languages and has traveled all over the world. She led a women's tour to China in 1984, and to India and Nepal in 1985. As a journalist accredited to the United Nations, she has reported from all United Nations women's, population, and Habitat conferences, and has addressed many international meetings and seminars.

For many years she has lectured widely on women's development and Female Genital Mutilation as well as urban development in the US, Europe and Africa, and has participated in many international conferences including all recent Inter-African Committee (IAC) conferences.

Women's International Network is a nonprofit organization registered in Massachusetts and has 501(c)3 status. Contributions are tax-deductible in the USA.

RESOURCES AND CONTACTS

The INTER-AFRICAN COMMITTEE (IAC) on Traditional Practices:
> c/o Economic Commission of Africa: P.O. Box 3001, Addis Ababa, Ethiopia
> Liaison Office: 147, rue de Lausanne, CH-1202 Geneva, Switzerland

A list of the **IAC affiliated groups** and addresses in 25 African countries is available. The IAC sponsors regional conferences every three years. The IAC has a Plan of Action and sponsors training and information campaigns in Africa. A videotape reports on activities. Teaching materials, visual aids and an anatomical model on FGM are available.

WIN NEWS: 187 Grant St., Lexington, MA 02173 USA - (617) 862-9431.
Quarterly journal about women and development; provides names/ contacts; reports on women's status and activities from more than 100 countries, including news on FGM.

WIN NEWS publishes: **The Childbirth Picture Books** in English / French / Arabic /Somali
> Additions to Prevent Excision and Infibulation // Flip Charts and Color Slides
> Free copies including the Additions for local groups in African countries where
> FGM is practiced as well as nonprofit groups working to stop FGM.

WIN NEWS also distributes FGM fact sheets, statistics, press releases, reprints of articles on FGM, lecture outlines and other information.

The HOSKEN REPORT: Genital and Sexual Mutilation of Females (fourth edition 1994), includes a bibliography and a global overview of FGM. 448 pp.